Machine Learning and Other Artificial Intelligence Applications

Editor

REZA FORGHANI

NEUROIMAGING CLINICS
OF NORTH AMERICA

www.neuroimaging.theclinics.com

Consulting Editor
SURESH K. MUKHERJI

November 2020 • Volume 30 • Number 4

ELSEVIER

1600 John F. Kennedy Boulevard ● Suite 1800 ● Philadelphia, Pennsylvania, 19103-2899

http://www.neuroimaging.theclinics.com

NEUROIMAGING CLINICS OF NORTH AMERICA Volume 30, Number 4
November 2020 ISSN 1052-5149, ISBN 13: 978-0-323-71244-6

Editor: John Vassallo (j.vassallo@elsevier.com)
Developmental Editor: Casey Potter

Neuroimaging Clinics of North America (ISSN 1052-5149) is published quarterly by Elsevier Inc., 360 Park Avenue South, New York, NY 10010-1710. Months of issue are February, May, August, and November. Business and editorial offices: 1600 John F. Kennedy Blvd., Suite 1800, Philadelphia, PA 19103-2899. Business and editorial offices: 6277 Sea Harbor Drive, Orlando, FL 32887-4800. Periodicals postage paid at New York, NY, and additional mailing offices. Subscription prices are USD 397 per year for US individuals, USD 686 per year for US institutions, USD 100 per year for US students and residents, USD 451 per year for Canadian individuals, USD 874 per year for Canadian institutions, USD 541 per year for international individuals, USD 874 per year for international institutions, USD 100 per year for Canadian students and residents and USD 260 per year for foreign students and residents. To receive student/resident rate, orders must be accompanied by name of affiliated institution, date of term, and the *signature* of program/residency coordinator on institution letterhead. Orders will be billed at individual rate until proof of status is received. Foreign air speed delivery is included in all *Clinics* subscription prices. All prices are subject to change without notice. POSTMASTER: Send address changes to *Neuroimaging Clinics of North America*, Elsevier Health Sciences Division, Subscription **Customer Service, 3251 Riverport Lane, Maryland Heights, MO 63043. Telephone: 1-800-654-2452 (U.S. and Canada); 314-447-8871 (outside U.S. and Canada). Fax: 314-447-8029. E-mail: journalscustomerservice-usa@elsevier.com (for print support); journalsonlinesupport-usa@elsevier.com (for online support).**

Reprints. For copies of 100 or more of articles in this publication, please contact the Commercial Reprints Department, Elsevier Inc., 360 Park Avenue South, New York, NY 10010-1710. Tel.: 212-633-3874; Fax: 212-633-3820; E-mail: reprints@elsevier.com.

Neuroimaging Clinics of North America is covered by *Excerpta Medical/EMBASE,* the RSNA Index of Imaging Literature, *MEDLINE/PubMed (Index Medicus),* MEDLINE/MEDLARS, SciSearch, Research Alert, and Neuroscience Citation Index.

PROGRAM OBJECTIVE

The goal of *Neuroimaging Clinics of North America* is to keep practicing radiologists and radiology residents up to date with current clinical practice in radiology by providing timely articles reviewing the state of the art in patient care.

TARGET AUDIENCE

Practicing radiologists, radiology residents, and other healthcare professionals who utilize neuroimaging findings to provide patient care.

LEARNING OBJECTIVES

Upon completion of this activity, participants will be able to:

1. Review various clinical applications of artificial intelligence (AI) in neurologic and head and neck imaging.
2. Discuss ethical and legal considerations of AI technology in imaging.
3. Recognize future role AI may play in enabling precise personalized therapy as part of a wholistic patient-centric care pathway.

ACCREDITATION

The Elsevier Office of Continuing Medical Education (EOCME) is accredited by the Accreditation Council for Continuing Medical Education (ACCME) to provide continuing medical education for physicians.

The EOCME designates this journal-based CME activity for a maximum of 13 *AMA PRA Category 1 Credit*(s)™. Physicians should claim only the credit commensurate with the extent of their participation in the activity.

All other healthcare professionals requesting continuing education credit for this enduring material will be issued a certificate of participation.

DISCLOSURE OF CONFLICTS OF INTEREST

The EOCME assesses conflict of interest with its instructors, faculty, planners, and other individuals who are in a position to control the content of CME activities. All relevant conflicts of interest that are identified are thoroughly vetted by EOCME for fair balance, scientific objectivity, and patient care recommendations. EOCME is committed to providing its learners with CME activities that promote improvements or quality in healthcare and not a specific proprietary business or a commercial interest.

The planning committee, staff, authors and editors listed below have identified no financial relationships or relationships to products or devices they or their spouse/life partner have with commercial interest related to the content of this CME activity:

John A. Boockvar, MD; David Camirand; Regina Chavous-Gibson, MSN, RN; Hui Chen, MD, PhD; Jaron J.R. Chong, MD, MHI, FRCPC; Michael Tran Duong, BA; Tobias D. Faizy, MD, PhD; Behzad Forghani, MEng; Reza Forghani, MD, PhD, FRCP(C), DABR; R. Gilberto Gonzalez, MD, PhD; Francois Guilbert, MD; Rajiv Gupta, MD, PhD; Jeremy J. Heit, MD, PhD; Bin Jiang, MD, PhD; Samuel Kadoury, PhD; Deepak Khatri, MD; Sanjith Prahas Krishnam, MBBS; Pradeep Kuttysankaran; William Trung Le, BSc; Laurent Letourneau-Guillon, MD, MSc; Michael H. Lev, MD; Jack W. Luo, MDCM; Farhad Maleki, PhD; Diego Martin, MD, PhD; Suresh K. Mukherji, MD, MBA, FACR; Nikesh Muthukrishnan, MEng; Keyhan Najafian, MSc; Katie Ovens, PhD; Andreas M. Rauschecker, MD, PhD; Caroline Reinhold, MD, MSc; Francisco Perdigón Romero, MSc; Thiparom Sananmuang, MD; Peter Savadjiev, PhD; Pamela W. Schaefer, MD; Elizabeth Tong, MD, PhD; John Vassallo; Yuan Xie, PhD; Guangming Zhu, MD, PhD; Avraham Zlochower, MD

The planning committee, staff, authors and editors listed below have identified financial relationships or relationships to products or devices they or their spouse/life partner have with commercial interest related to the content of this CME activity:

Peter D. Chang, MD: owns stock and holds patents with Avicenna.AI and is a consultant/advisor, on a speakers bureau, and receives research support from Canon Medical Systems, USA

Daniel S. Chow, MD: owns stock in Avicenna.AI and is a consultant/advisor for Canon Medical Systems, USA

Christopher G. Filippi, MD: owns stock in Avicenna.AI

Suyash Mohan, MD: receives research support from Galileo, Inc. and Novocure

Max Wintermark, MD, MAS: owns equity interest in Subtle Medical, Inc

Greg Zaharchuk, MD, PhD: owns equity interest in Subtle Medical, Inc

UNAPPROVED/OFF-LABEL USE DISCLOSURE

The EOCME requires CME faculty to disclose to the participants:

1. When products or procedures being discussed are off-label, unlabelled, experimental, and/or investigational (not US Food and Drug Administration [FDA] approved); and
2. Any limitations on the information presented, such as data that are preliminary or that represent ongoing research, interim analyses, and/or unsupported opinions. Faculty may discuss information about pharmaceutical agents that is outside of FDA-approved labelling. This information is intended solely for CME and is not intended to promote off-label use of these

medications. If you have any questions, contact the medical affairs department of the manufacturer for the most recent pre-scribing information.

TO ENROLL
To enroll in the *Neuroimaging Clinics of North America* Continuing Medical Education program, call customer service at 1-800-654-2452 or sign up online at http://www.theclinics.com/home/cme. The CME program is available to subscribers for an additional annual fee of USD 245.00.

METHOD OF PARTICIPATION
In order to claim credit, participants must complete the following:
1. Complete enrolment as indicated above.
2. Read the activity.
3. Complete the CME Test and Evaluation. Participants must achieve a score of 70% on the test. All CME Tests and Evaluations must be completed online.

CME INQUIRIES/SPECIAL NEEDS
For all CME inquiries or special needs, please contact elsevierCME@elsevier.com.

NEUROIMAGING CLINICS OF NORTH AMERICA

THE CLINICS ARE AVAILABLE ONLINE!
Access your subscription at:
www.theclinics.com

NEUROIMAGING CLINICS OF NORTH AMERICA

Contributors

CONSULTING EDITOR

SURESH K. MUKHERJI, MD, MBA, FACR
Clinical Professor, Marian University, Director
of Head and Neck Radiology, ProScan
Imaging, Regional Medical Director, Envision
Physician Services, Carmel, Indiana, USA

EDITOR

REZA FORGHANI, MD, PhD, FRCP(C), DABR
Associate Professor, Department of Radiology,
McGill University and McGill University Health
Centre, Director and Lead Investigator,
Augmented Intelligence & Precision Health
Laboratory (AIPHL) of the Department of
Radiology and the Research Institute of McGill
University Health Centre (RI MUHC), FRQS
Clinical Research Scholar (Chercheur-Boursier
Clinicien) and Clinical Investigator, RI MUHC,
Segal Cancer Centre and Lady Davis Research

Institute of the Jewish General Hospital,
Associate Member, McGill University
Department of Otolaryngology - Head and
Neck Surgery and Gerald Bronfman
Department of Oncology, Theme Leader,
Artificial Intelligence-Assisted Radiomics for
Advanced Diagnostics, McGill Centre for
Translational Research in Cancer, Director,
Combined Clinical-Research Head and Neck
Imaging Fellowship, Montreal, Quebec,
Canada

AUTHORS

JOHN A. BOOCKVAR, MD
Vice Chair of Neurosurgery, Professor,
Department of Neurosurgery, Lenox Hill
Hospital, Donald and Barbara Zucker School of
Medicine at Hofstra/Northwell, New York, New
York, USA

DAVID CAMIRAND
Department of Radiology, Centre Hospitalier
de l'Université de Montréal (CHUM), Montréal,
Québec, Canada

PETER D. CHANG, MD
Assistant Professor, Department of Radiology,
University of California-Irvine School of
Medicine, Co-Director, Center for Artificial
Intelligence in Diagnostic Medicine (CAIDM),
Orange, California, USA

HUI CHEN, MD, PhD
Department of Neuroradiology, Stanford
University, Stanford, California, USA

JARON J.R. CHONG, MD, MHI, FRCPC
Department of Medical Imaging, Western
University, London, Ontario, Canada

DANIEL S. CHOW, MD
Assistant Professor, Department of Radiology,
University of California-Irvine School of
Medicine, Co-Director, Center for Artificial
Intelligence in Diagnostic Medicine (CAIDM),
Orange, California, USA

MICHAEL TRAN DUONG, BA
Department of Radiology, Perelman School of
Medicine at the University of Pennsylvania,
Philadelphia, Pennsylvania, USA

TOBIAS D. FAIZY, MD, PhD
Department of Neuroradiology, Stanford
University, Stanford, California, USA

CHRISTOPHER G. FILIPPI, MD
Vice Chair, Biomedical Imaging and
Translational Science, Professor, Department

of Radiology, Lenox Hill Hospital, Donald and Barbara Zucker School of Medicine at Hofstra/Northwell, New York, New York, USA

BEHZAD FORGHANI, MEng
Augmented Intelligence & Precision Health Laboratory (AIPHL), Department of Radiology and Research Institute of the McGill University Health Centre, Gerald Bronfman Department of Oncology, McGill University, Montreal, Quebec, Canada

REZA FORGHANI, MD, PhD, FRCP(C), DABR
Associate Professor, Department of Radiology, McGill University and McGill University Health Centre, Director and Lead Investigator, Augmented Intelligence & Precision Health Laboratory (AIPHL) of the Department of Radiology and the Research Institute of McGill University Health Centre (RI MUHC), FRQS Clinical Research Scholar (Chercheur-Boursier Clinicien) and Clinical Investigator, RI MUHC, Segal Cancer Centre and Lady Davis Research Institute of the Jewish General Hospital, Associate Member, McGill University Department of Otolaryngology - Head and Neck Surgery and Gerald Bronfman Department of Oncology, Theme Leader, Artificial Intelligence-Assisted Radiomics for Advanced Diagnostics, McGill Centre for Translational Research in Cancer, Director, Combined Clinical-Research Head and Neck Imaging Fellowship, Montreal, Quebec, Canada; 4intelligent Inc., Cote St-Luc, Quebec, Canada

R. GILBERTO GONZALEZ, MD, PhD
Division Chief and Professor, Department of Radiology, Division of Neuroradiology, Massachusetts General Hospital, Harvard Medical School, Boston, Massachusetts, USA

FRANCOIS GUILBERT, MD
Department of Radiology, Centre Hospitalier de l'Université de Montréal (CHUM), Centre de Recherche du CHUM (CRCHUM), Montréal, Québec, Canada

RAJIV GUPTA, MD, PhD
Associate Radiologist, Associate Professor, Department of Radiology, Division of Neuroradiology, Massachusetts General Hospital, Harvard Medical School, Boston, Massachusetts, USA

JEREMY J. HEIT, MD, PhD
Department of Neuroradiology, Stanford University, Stanford, California, USA

BIN JIANG, MD, PhD
Department of Neuroradiology, Stanford University, Stanford, California, USA

SAMUEL KADOURY, PhD
Polytechnique Montreal, CHUM Research Center, Montreal, Quebec, Canada

DEEPAK KHATRI, MD
Neurosurgery Resident, Department of Neurosurgery, Lenox Hill Hospital, Donald and Barbara Zucker School of Medicine at Hofstra/Northwell, New York, New York, USA

SANJITH PRAHAS KRISHNAM, MBBS
Resident Physician, Department of Neurology, University of Alabama at Birmingham, Birmingham, Alabama, USA

WILLIAM TRUNG LE, BSc
Polytechnique Montreal, CHUM Research Center, Montreal, Quebec, Canada

LAURENT LETOURNEAU-GUILLON, MD, MSc
Department of Radiology, Centre Hospitalier de l'Université de Montréal (CHUM), Centre de Recherche du CHUM (CRCHUM), Montréal, Québec, Canada

MICHAEL H. LEV, MD
Division Chief and Professor, Department of Radiology, Division of Emergency Radiology, Massachusetts General Hospital, Harvard Medical School, Department of Radiology, Division of Neuroradiology, Massachusetts General Hospital, Boston, Massachusetts, USA

JACK W. LUO, MDCM
Department of Radiology, McGill University, Montreal, Quebec, Canada

FARHAD MALEKI, PhD
Augmented Intelligence & Precision Health Laboratory (AIPHL), Department of Radiology and Research Institute of the McGill University Health Centre, Montreal, Quebec, Canada

DIEGO MARTIN, MD, PhD
Department of Diagnostic Radiology, McGill University, Augmented Intelligence & Precision Health Laboratory (AIPHL), Department of Diagnostic Radiology, Research Institute of the McGill University Health Centre, Montreal, Quebec, Canada

SUYASH MOHAN, MD
Associate Professor of Radiology and Neurosurgery, Department of Radiology, Perelman School of Medicine at the University of Pennsylvania, Philadelphia, Pennsylvania, USA

NIKESH MUTHUKRISHNAN, MEng
Augmented Intelligence & Precision Health Laboratory (AIPHL), Department of Radiology & Research Institute of the McGill University Health Centre, Montreal, Quebec, Canada

KEYHAN NAJAFIAN, MSc
Augmented Intelligence & Precision Health Laboratory (AIPHL), Research Institute of the McGill University Health Centre, Montreal, Quebec, Canada

KATIE OVENS, PhD
Augmented Intelligence & Precision Health Laboratory (AIPHL), Department of Radiology & Research Institute of the McGill University Health Centre, Montreal, Quebec, Canada; University of Saskatchewan, Saskatoon, Saskatchewan, Canada

ANDREAS M. RAUSCHECKER, MD, PhD
Assistant Professor, Department of Radiology & Biomedical Imaging, University of California, San Francisco, San Francisco, California, USA

CAROLINE REINHOLD, MD, MSc
Augmented Intelligence & Precision Health Laboratory (AIPHL), Department of Radiology and Research Institute of the McGill University Health Centre, Department of Radiology, McGill University, Department of Diagnostic Radiology, Research Institute of the McGill University Health Centre, Montreal, Quebec, Canada

FRANCISCO PERDIGÓN ROMERO, MSc
Polytechnique Montreal, Montreal, Quebec, Canada

THIPAROM SANANMUANG, MD
Department of Diagnostic and Therapeutic Radiology and Research, Faculty of Medicine Ramathibodi Hospital, Ratchathewi, Bangkok, Thailand

PETER SAVADJIEV, PhD
Department of Diagnostic Radiology, McGill University, School of Computer Science, McGill University, Medical Physics Unit, Department of Oncology, McGill University, Augmented Intelligence & Precision Health Laboratory (AIPHL), Department of Diagnostic Radiology, Research Institute of the McGill University Health Centre, Montreal, Quebec, Canada

PAMELA W. SCHAEFER, MD
Vice-Chair and Professor, Department of Radiology, Division of Neuroradiology, Massachusetts General Hospital, Harvard Medical School, Boston, Massachusetts, USA

ELIZABETH TONG, MD, PhD
Department of Neuroradiology, Stanford University, Stanford, California, USA

MAX WINTERMARK, MD, MAS
Department of Neuroradiology, Stanford University, Stanford, California, USA

YUAN XIE, PhD
Department of Neuroradiology, Stanford University, Stanford, California, USA

GREG ZAHARCHUK, MD, PhD
Department of Neuroradiology, Stanford University, Stanford, California, USA

GUANGMING ZHU, MD, PhD
Department of Neuroradiology, Stanford University, Stanford, California, USA

AVRAHAM ZLOCHOWER, MD
Assistant Professor, Department of Radiology, Lenox Hill Hospital, Donald and Barbara Zucker School of Medicine at Hofstra/Northwell, New York, New York, USA

DIEGO MARTIN, MD, PhD
Department of Diagnostic Radiology, McGill University, Augmented Intelligence & Precision Health Laboratory (AIPHL), Department of Diagnostic Radiology, Research Institute of the McGill University Health Centre, Montreal, Quebec, Canada

SUYASH MOHAN, MD
Associate Professor of Radiology and Neurosurgery, Department of Radiology, Perelman School of Medicine at the University of Pennsylvania, Philadelphia, Pennsylvania, USA

NIKESH MUTHUKRISHNAN, MEng
Augmented Intelligence & Precision Health Laboratory (AIPHL), Department of Radiology & Research Institute of the McGill University Health Centre, Montreal, Quebec, Canada

KEYHAN NAJAFIAN, MSc
Augmented Intelligence & Precision Health Laboratory (AIPHL), Research Institute of the McGill University Health Centre, Montreal, Quebec, Canada

KATIE OVENS, PhD
Augmented Intelligence & Precision Health Laboratory (AIPHL), Department of Radiology & Research Institute of the McGill University Health Centre, Montreal, Quebec, Canada, University of Saskatchewan, Saskatoon, Saskatchewan, Canada

ANDREAS M. RAUSCHECKER, MD, PhD
Assistant Professor, Department of Radiology & Biomedical Imaging, University of California, San Francisco, San Francisco, California, USA

CAROLINE REINHOLD, MD, MSc
Augmented Intelligence & Precision Health Laboratory (AIPHL), Department of Radiology and Research Institute of the McGill University Health Centre, Department of Radiology, McGill University, Department of Diagnostic Radiology, Research Institute of the McGill University Health Centre, Montreal, Quebec, Canada

FRANCISCO PERDIGÓN ROMERO, MSc
Polytechnique Montreal, Montreal, Quebec, Canada

THIRAROM SANANMUANG, MD
Department of Diagnostic and Therapeutic Radiology and Research, Faculty of Medicine, Ramathibodi Hospital, Ratchathewi, Bangkok, Thailand

PETER SAVADJIEV, PhD
Department of Diagnostic Radiology, McGill University, School of Computer Science, McGill University, Medical Physics Unit, Department of Oncology, McGill University, Augmented Intelligence & Precision Health Laboratory (AIPHL), Department of Diagnostic Radiology, Research Institute of the McGill University Health Centre, Montreal, Quebec, Canada

PAMELA A. W. SCHAEFER, MD
Vice-Chair and Professor, Department of Radiology, Division of Neuroradiology, Massachusetts General Hospital, Harvard Medical School, Boston, Massachusetts, USA

ELIZABETH TONG, MD, PhD
Department of Neuroradiology, Stanford University, Stanford, California, USA

MAX WINTERMARK, MD, MAS
Department of Neuroradiology, Stanford University, Stanford, California, USA

YUAN XIE, PhD
Department of Neuroradiology, Stanford University, Stanford, California, USA

GREG ZAHARCHUK, MD, PhD
Department of Neuroradiology, Stanford University, Stanford, California, USA

GUANGMING ZHU, MD, PhD
Department of Neuroradiology, Stanford University, Stanford, California, USA

AVRAHAM ZLOCHOWER, MD
Assistant Professor, Department of Radiology, Lenox Hill Hospital, Donald and Barbara Zucker School of Medicine at Hofstra/Northwell, New York, New York, USA

Contents

early imaging, alert care teams, and assist in treatment selection. This article reviews algorithms for artificial intelligence techniques that may be used to detect and localize acute ischemic stroke. We describe artificial intelligence algorithms for these tasks and illustrate them with examples.

Artificial intelligence (AI) advancements have significant implications for medical imaging. Stroke is the leading cause of disability and the fifth leading cause of death in the United States. AI applications for stroke imaging are a topic of intense research. AI techniques are well-suited for dealing with vast amounts of stroke imaging data and a large number of multidisciplinary approaches used in classification, risk assessment, segmentation tasks, diagnosis, prognosis, and even prediction of therapy responses. This article addresses this topic and seeks to present an overview of machine learning and/or deep learning applied to stroke imaging.

Deep learning represents end-to-end machine learning in which feature selection from images and classification happen concurrently. This articles provides updates on how deep learning is being applied to the study of glioma and its genetic heterogeneity. Deep learning algorithms can detect patterns in routine and advanced MR imaging that elude the eyes of neuroradiologists and make predictions about glioma genetics, which impact diagnosis, treatment response, patient management, and long-term survival. The success of these deep learning initiatives may enhance the performance of neuroradiologists and add greater value to patient care by expediting treatment.

Recent advances in artificial intelligence (AI) and deep learning (DL) hold promise to augment neuroimaging diagnosis for patients with brain tumors and stroke. Here, the authors review the diverse landscape of emerging neuroimaging applications of AI, including workflow optimization, lesion segmentation, and precision education. Given the many modalities used in diagnosing neurologic diseases, AI may be deployed to integrate across modalities (MR imaging, computed tomography, PET, electroencephalography, clinical and laboratory findings), facilitate crosstalk among specialists, and potentially improve diagnosis in patients with trauma, multiple sclerosis, epilepsy, and neurodegeneration. Together, there are myriad applications of AI for neuroradiology.

The head and neck (HN) consists of a large number of vital anatomic structures within a compact area. Imaging plays a central role in the diagnosis and management of major disorders affecting the HN. This article reviews the recent applications of machine learning (ML) in HN imaging with a focus on deep learning approaches. It categorizes ML applications in HN imaging into deep learning and traditional ML applications and provides examples of each category. It also discusses the main challenges facing the successful deployment of ML-based applications in the clinical setting and provides suggestions for addressing these challenges.

Online Only Articles, available at www.neuroimaging. theclinics.com, ScienceDirect, and ClinicalKey

There is great potential for artificial intelligence (AI) applications, especially machine learning and natural language processing, in medical imaging. Much attention has been garnered by the image analysis tasks for diagnostic decision support and precision medicine, but there are many other potential applications of AI in radiology and have potential to enhance all levels of the radiology workflow and practice, including workflow optimization and support for interpretation tasks, quality and safety, and operational efficiency. This article reviews the important potential applications of informatics and AI related to process improvement and operations in the radiology department.

The extensive body of research and advances in machine learning (ML) and the availability of a large volume of patient data make ML a powerful tool for producing models with the potential for widespread deployment in clinical settings. This article provides an overview of the classic supervised and unsupervised ML methods as well as fundamental concepts required for understanding how to develop generalizable and high-performing ML applications. It also describes the important steps for developing a ML model and how decisions made in these steps affect model performance and ability to generalize.

Foreword

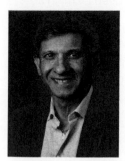

Suresh K. Mukherji, MD, MBA, FACR
Consulting Editor

Artificial Intelligence (AI)… What is it? …How does it work? …How good is it? …How can it help us? …Will it replace us? ☹ These questions inspired us to devote an issue of *Neuroimaging Clinics* to this important topic. AI is already part of our daily lives, and this issue attempts to answer these and more regarding how augmenting human intelligence will impact the field of Radiology…and us!

This issue has beautifully written articles covering the history of AI, review of techniques, clinical applications in neuroradiology, and role of AI in quality improvement. There is also an article devoted to ethical and legal considerations of AI. The roster of article authors is impressive and comprises a "Who's Who" in this dynamic field. I also would like to express my deepest gratitude to the authors for their wonderful contributions.

Finally, I would like to thank my friend and colleague, Dr Reza Forghani, MD, PhD, FRCP(C),

DABR, for agreeing to edit this important issue. Reza is one of the most talented, dynamic, and energetic individuals I have ever met. I always felt the world could solve all of its "fossil fuel" issues if we could somehow "tap" into Reza's unbridled energy. ☺ Thank you very much, Reza, for all you do on so many levels!

Suresh K. Mukherji, MD, MBA, FACR
Clinical Professor, Marian University
Director of Head and Neck Radiology
ProScan Imaging
Regional Medical Director
Envision Physician Services
Carmel, Indiana, USA

E-mail address:
sureshmukherji@hotmail.com

https://doi.org/10.1016/j.nic.2020.08.005
1052-5149/20/© 2020 Published by Elsevier Inc.

Preface
Machine Intelligence in Neurologic and Head and Neck Imaging

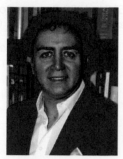

Reza Forghani, MD, PhD, FRCP(C), DABR
Editor

Interest in intelligent machines is not new, and serious attempts at building machines that can solve problems and make decisions simulating what humans do were already underway in the 1950s. However, the field of artificial intelligence (AI) has clearly seen a revolutionary revival in the last decade. This is at least in part fueled by developments in application of deep neural networks for complex analytic and image analysis tasks, made possible by the impressive progress and achievements in hardware development and computing power. AI is already incorporated in our daily lives. As a testament, one must look no further than at smart phones, commonly used search engines, social media, or smart home devices. There is also increasing adoption in various major industries. Not surprisingly, there is a lot of interest in health care applications, especially in imaging, where the core data (ie, medical images) have been in digital format for many years and therefore optimally stored and available for computerized analysis and AI applications.

There is no doubt that this disruptive technology has the potential to reshape health care in the long term. However, at least in the foreseeable future, AI's application potential is not unlimited. Extreme scenarios of AI representing a be-all and end-all solution and replacement for everything not only are unrealistic but also do disservice to the technology by setting unrealistic

expectations that could inevitably lead to disappointment, in addition to hindering engagement by the very professionals with the domain knowledge needed to successfully implement AI in the clinical setting. At the same time, most experts would agree that ignoring this technology would be at one's own peril, and it is imperative for physicians to leverage this technology to improve health care processes. The purpose of this issue is to familiarize radiologists and other health care professionals, who are interested in neurologic and head and neck imaging, with the strengths and limitations of AI technology and its potential positive impact in improving the health care enterprise by augmenting human intelligence.

This issue consists of a collection of review articles written by experts across North America that includes general technical reviews, reviews of various clinical applications in neurologic and head and neck imaging, and reviews related to the use of AI for process improvement and incorporation in smart devices. In addition to discussing current proposed image-based applications, this collection is meant to provide a glimpse into the future, as this disruptive technology is likely to blur traditional specialty boundaries and integrate different information in order to enable precise personalized therapy as part of a wholistic patient-centric care pathway. It is my hope that

1052-5149/20/© 2020 Published by Elsevier Inc.

neuroimaging.theclinics.com

the content can serve as a resource and catalyst both for those unfamiliar and for those already entrenched in AI research or clinical implementation.

I conclude by expressing my gratitude to Dr Suresh K. Mukherji for the opportunity to guest edit this issue of *Neuroimaging Clinics* and by thanking all the authors for their fantastic work and contributions to this issue. This issue would not have been possible without the support and patience of John Vassallo, Associate Publisher, and Casey Potter and Nicholas Henderson, Developmental Editors at Elsevier. I hope that our readers will find the issue both informative and inspiring.

Reza Forghani, MD, PhD, FRCP(C), DABR
McGill University Health Centre
Department of Radiology
Augmented Intelligence &
Precision Health Laboratory (AIPHL)
C02.5821, 1001 Decarie Boulevard
Montreal, Quebec H4A 3J1, Canada

E-mail address:
reza.forghani@mcgill.ca

Brief History of Artificial Intelligence

Nikesh Muthukrishnan, MEng[a], Farhad Maleki, PhD[a], Katie Ovens, PhD[a,b],
Caroline Reinhold, MD, MSc[a,c], Behzad Forghani, MEng[a,d], Reza Forghani, MD, PhD[a,c,d,e,f],*

KEYWORDS

- Artificial intelligence • History • AI winter • Neural network • Convolutional neural network
- Machine learning • Deep learning

KEY POINTS

- There have been several cycles in the past 70 years where artificial intelligence has showed great promise and eventually failed to meet its high expectations.
- Failure to meet expectations owing to limitations of artificial intelligence causes a loss of interest by public and stakeholders.
- These failures have forced the field of artificial intelligence into "artificial intelligence winters," where growth is severely reduced.
- Although the most recent advances in artificial intelligence and successes in deep learning are promising, artificial intelligence has limitations.
- There should realistic expectations set to avoid a third artificial intelligence winter.

INTRODUCTION

Artificial intelligence (AI) is revolutionizing many industries by performing tasks that typically require human intelligence to solve. AI contributes to complex scientific and engineering workflows through simulating, supplementing, or augmenting human intelligence in an efficient and precise manner. Examples of such tasks include fraud detection in banking, conversational bots used in customer service, and precision diagnostics in health care. AI aims at programming intelligence into machines by learning from experiences and adapting to changes in the environment to simulate human decision making and reasoning processes.

Machine learning (ML), a subfield of AI (**Fig. 1**), is concerned with algorithms that are capable of learning complex tasks and developing predictive models through sample data. Through a procedure referred to as feature engineering, often a set of informative features are selected or generated by an expert for building predictive models. The availability of large amounts of data and computational power has led to a surge in successful

Funding Information: R. Forghani is a clinical research scholar (chercheur-boursier clinicien) supported by the Fonds de recherche en santé du Québec (FRQS) and has an operating grant jointly funded by the FRQS and the Fondation de l'Association des radiologistes du Québec (FARQ).

[a] Augmented Intelligence & Precision Health Laboratory (AIPHL), Department of Radiology & Research Institute of the McGill University Health Centre, 5252 Boulevard de Maisonneuve Ouest, Montreal, Quebec H4A 3S5, Canada; [b] University of Saskatchewan, 116 - 110 Science Place, Saskatoon, SK S7N 5C9, Canada; [c] Department of Radiology, McGill University, 1650 Cedar Avenue, Montreal, Quebec H3G 1A4, Canada; [d] Gerald Bronfman Department of Oncology, McGill University, Suite 720, 5100 Maisonneuve Boulevard West, Montreal, Quebec H4A3T2, Canada; [e] Segal Cancer Centre, Lady Davis Institute for Medical Research, Jewish General Hospital, 3755 Cote Ste-Catherine Road, Montreal, Quebec H3T 1E2, Canada; [f] Department of Otolaryngology - Head and Neck Surgery, Royal Victoria Hospital, McGill University Health Centre, 1001 boul. Decarie Boulevard, Montreal, Quebec H3A 3J1, Canada

* Corresponding author. Room C02.5821, 1001 Decarie Boulevard, Montreal, Quebec H4A 3J1, Canada.
E-mail address: reza.forghani@mcgill.ca

Neuroimag Clin N Am 30 (2020) 393–399
https://doi.org/10.1016/j.nic.2020.07.004
1052-5149/20/

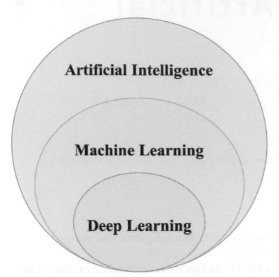

Fig. 1. AI aims at simulating human intelligence. ML, a subfield of AI, is concerned with learning complex associations using data. ML methodologies focus on developing predictive models using sample data. Through a process referred to as feature engineering, human experts select informative features to build predictive models. DL, which is a subfield of ML, tries to eliminate the feature engineering step by learning the optimal set of features from sample data.

applications of ML in fields such as natural language processing, machine vision, robotics, and diagnostics.[1–4] Most of the recent successes in ML applications can be attributed to the advances and innovations in deep learning (DL), which is considered a subfield of ML. DL refers to the methodologies that rely on deep neural networks. DL methods eliminate the need for feature engineering by trying to learn the optimal set of features from data. Neural networks were initially designed to simulate neural activities in a human brain. As the development and interest in the field continues to expand, it is important to appreciate its history as well as understand the potential pitfalls.

EARLIEST ATTEMPTS AT ARTIFICIAL INTELLIGENCE

The earliest models of AI tried to simulate the function of a single neuron (**Fig. 2**). The simplest models started as feedforward, simple input–output functions. However, over the following decades, these became more sophisticated with the addition of more sophisticated functions, added layers, and bidirectional feedback, eventually becoming the building blocks of the modern day deep neural networks or DL. One of the first publications alluding to AI was work published by

McCulloch and Pitts in 1943.[5] Their publication describes a computer model used to learn based on a process comparable with neurons in the human brain. The model described in their publication was referred to as the MCP neuron, and it functioned by taking in Boolean inputs (Boolean logic refers to a branch of algebra concerning true/false statements), processing them in a preset manner, and if the processed value exceeded a certain threshold, the MCP neuron would output a value. By exceeding the threshold, the MCP neuron is considered to have been fired or activated. Although this simple model was effective for simple processing tasks, it had many limitations. It generated a binary output and required a fixed set of weight and threshold values. Also, they did not provide a methodology for learning those values.

A more sophisticated version of the MCP was published in 1958 by Rosenblatt, called the perceptron.[6] The perceptron, illustrated in (**Fig. 3**) processed non-Boolean inputs $(x_1, x_2, \cdots, x_n)$ and included weights into the model $(w_1, w_2, \cdots, w_n)$ for scaling. In addition, a nonlinear function f processes the sum of the products of the input values and their corresponding weights. This provided more flexibility to the model and later became one of the building blocks for modern neural networks.

With increased development of early AI models and the inevitable progress in the field, a systematic methodology for evaluating the intelligence of a model was necessary. One of the first works introducing the topic of a model's intelligence was published by Alan Turing, entitled "Computing Machinery and Intelligence," in October 1950.[7] Turing raised the question of whether machines can imitate human intelligence and introduced a test for model intelligence. This test, referred to as the Turing Test, involves a blinded human interrogator questioning a human respondent and a machine respondent. The task of the interrogator is to identify which respondent is the machine. If the interrogator is not capable of discerning the machine answers from the human answers more often that what would be expected by chance, the machine is considered to have passed the Turing Test. The Turing Test has typically been considered the goal of AI; however, in modern days, there is a debate on whether the Turing Test distracts AI researchers in addition to unnecessarily raising the public expectation of the field.[8] The 1956 Dartmouth conference is generally considered the moment that AI formally recognized and obtained its name and its mission.[9,10] This conference was organized by Marvin Minsky, John McCarthy, Claude Shannon, and Nathan

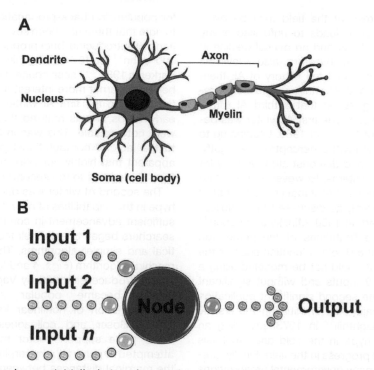

Fig. 2. Neural networks were initially designed to simulate neurons in the human brain (*A*), composed of artificial neurons or nodes (*B*). A node has an activation function, defining the output of that node based on an input or set of inputs. Although in their earliest forms these had feedforward, simple input–output functions, overtime these became more sophisticated, eventually becoming the building blocks of the modern day deep neural networks (see text for additional details). An example of a neural network neuron is depicted in 2B.

Rochester of IBM and may be considered the "birth" of the field of AI, including the assertion that "every aspect of learning or any other feature of intelligence can be so precisely described that a machine can be made to simulate it."

CYCLES OF INTEREST IN ARTIFICIAL INTELLIGENCE AND THE FIRST AND SECOND ARTIFICIAL INTELLIGENCE WINTERS

With media coverage and public expectations being high, AI can often be overhyped, and the slow

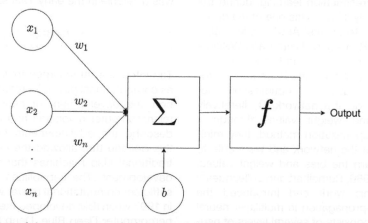

Fig. 3. A visualization of the perceptron, which is one of the building blocks of modern neural networks. A perceptron is a mathematical model for a biological neuron. It takes input values (x_1, x_2, $\cdots$,x_n), weight values of (w_1, w_2, $\cdots$,w_n), and a bias value of b. First, each input value is multiplied by its corresponding weight; then the summation of the resulting values and the bias value is calculated to generate a single value. This value is then fed to a function f, referred to as an activation function. The activation function generates a binary value, that is, 0 or 1, depending on its input. This model can be used as a binary classifier.

but steady progress of the field may be overlooked. This situation leads to unfulfilled overly ambitious expectations and an overall decline in interest in the field by investors, also known as an AI winter. Throughout the history of AI, there have already been 2 AI winters, and some researchers are suggesting that a third AI winter may be arriving soon. The first AI winter was between the years of 1974 and 1980. Leading up to these years, Rosenblatt's perceptron had gathered a lot of hype and demonstrated capacity for modeling simple systems. However, the unrealistic initial expectations of AI at that time also started to become apparent, as discussed in 2 publications that emerged. In 1968, Minsky and Papert[11] demonstrated the limitations of the perceptron by identifying that a Boolean function such as the XOR function that could not be modeled using a perceptron with 2 inputs and without significant user handling. The second significant publication that played a major role in initiating the first AI winter was by Lighthill[12] in 1973, providing an overview of the hype in the field and emphasis on the very small progress in the field. Finally, during these years, many governmental organizations stopped funding for AI research or significantly decreased their AI research funding.[13] After 1980, most AI researchers had given up on AI algorithms learning representations of data and instead shifted toward expert rule-based systems. However, by the mid 1980s, it was recognized that, although expert systems were capable of performing very specific tasks, these models lacked common sense, could not be used to perform more complex tasks, and were not generalizable.[14]

The lack of representation learning, during the late 1970s and early 1980s, was one of the drawbacks that had led to the first AI winter. In 1985 a seminal work by Rumelhart, Hinton and Williams ended this long winter.[15] They addressed the concerns presented by Minsky and Papert and introduced gradient descent optimization for minimizing the error of a network. By iteratively updating bias and weight values through a gradient decent optimization method, they minimized the error of the network and were able to systematically learn the bias and weight values. Furthermore, in 1986, Rumelhart and colleagues[16] expanded on this work and introduced the concept of back-propagation in multilayer neural networks, which consists of several layers of neurons stacked together where neurons in each layer were connected to the neurons in the next layer. The back-propagation algorithm revolutionized the learning capabilities of neural networks. Although Rumelhart and colleagues were credited

for popularizing back-propagation, it is important to note that there had been several earlier publications of introducing backpropagation by Werbos and John[17] in 1974, Fukushima[18] in 1980, and Parker in 1985.[19] These concepts and publications began to garner more interest and funding for the field, ending the first AI winter. However, in the early 1990s, it was realized that these networks were not scalable. This was in large part related to the lack of computational power. It became apparent that highly complex networks were not feasible, leading to the second AI winter.

The second AI winter was due to the increased hype in the capabilities of neural networks without sufficient advancement in computing power. Researchers began to shift their focus to more practical and simpler algorithms. The support vector machine algorithm (**Figs. 4** and **5**), which was originally introduced in 1963 by Vapnik and Chervonenkis, became popular again with the implementation of nonlinear kernels in 1992.[20] Before Boser and colleagues' publication in 1992,[20] the support vector machine algorithm attempted to solve for a hyperplane by maximizing the marginal distances between 2 separate classes and the hyperplane. The maximized distance between the hyperplane and the classes allows for more robustness because data are always subject to noise. The publication by Boser allowed for a simple modification of the optimization algorithm, now known as the "kernel trick," which enabled the algorithm to solve for nonlinear hyperplanes without significantly increasing the computational requirements of the algorithm. This trick allowed for support vector machine algorithms to capitalize on the low computational power that was available in the early 1990s.

RESURGENCE OF INTEREST IN ARTIFICIAL INTELLIGENCE: THE THIRD WAVE

The interest in AI resurged toward the mid 1990s as computational power increased and could support the development of neural networks. The microcomputer revolution and Moore's law both describe the advancements computers had in this decade that allowed the replacement of the traditional Lisp machines that were throttling AI development. The capabilities of AI paired with sufficient computational power was demonstrated in 1997 when IBM developed the chess playing supercomputer Deep Blue. Deep Blue defeated the chess champion Kasparov, which led to many publications and documentary films that attracted the public's attention to the field once again.[21,22]

Neural networks began to resurface in the late 1990's with the introduction of convolutional

Support Vector Example

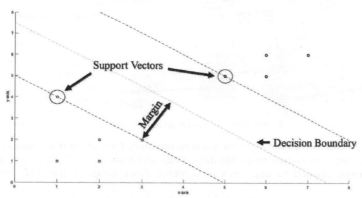

Fig. 4. Example of a support vector machine. (*From* Forghani R, Savadjiev P, Chatterjee A, et al. Radiomics and Artificial Intelligence for Biomarker and Prediction Model Development in Oncology. Comput Struct Biotechnol J. 2019;17:995-1008. Published 2019 Jul 12. https://doi.org/10.1016/j.csbj.2019.07.001; with permission.)

neural networks. LeCun and colleagues[23] published the LeNet-5 network (a 7-level convolutional neural network) in 1998 for document recognition, which used convolutional and subsampling layers processing the input before a fully connected layer for output prediction (**Fig. 6**). Although they were able to achieve the lowest error rates on digit recognition at that time, the algorithm had difficulties scaling to larger problems because they were limited by hardware and data constraints. This issue continued to plague the neural network algorithms for almost a decade. During the last decade, there were 2 main advancements that enabled neural networks to progress: data storage and graphical processing units (GPU). Data became more readily accessible with electronic storage and lower costs. The performance of ML algorithms relies heavily on the available data. Thus, with a high volume of available data, the performance of these algorithms improved. This development enabled the Hinton and colleagues'[24] laboratory to formally introduce DL to

the public in 2006 and achieve exceptional performance in speech recognition, which was previously determined to be a challenging AI problem.

Furthermore, with the introduction of GPUs and the steady improvement to computers as per Moore's law, the hardware limitations that constrained the performance of neural networks were overcome. The additional computational power enabled researchers to run larger networks with more complex layers. Cireşan and colleagues[25] were the first to implement GPUs with DL using a GTX 280 graphics card. Finally, in 2012, Krizhevsky and colleagues[26] presented AlexNet, which used the massively available dataset from ImageNet (1.2 million images with 1000 classes at the time) with GPUs to win the ImageNet Large Scale Visual Recognition Challenge. Krizhevsky and colleagues used the rectified linear units to introduce nonlinearities to convolutional neural networks as well as the dropout technique to avoid overfitting. AlexNet was able to achieve an error rate of 15.3% on the dataset, which was

Higher Order Transformation

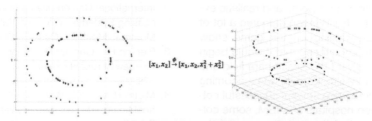

$$[x_1, x_2] \xrightarrow{\phi} [x_1, x_2, x_1^2 + x_2^2]$$

Fig. 5. Example of support vector machines: nonlinearly separable data transformed to a higher dimension. (*From* Forghani R, Savadjiev P, Chatterjee A, et al. Radiomics and Artificial Intelligence for Biomarker and Prediction Model Development in Oncology. Comput Struct Biotechnol J. 2019;17:995-1008. Published 2019 Jul 12. https://doi.org/10.1016/j.csbj.2019.07.001; with permission.)

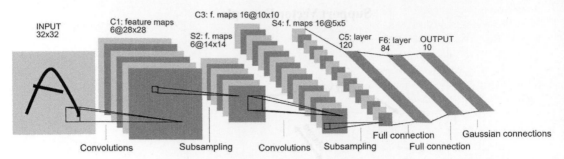

Fig. 6. Architecture of LeNet-5, a CNN, here for digits recognition. Each plane is a feature map, that is, a set of units whose weights are constrained to be identical. (*Adapted from* Lecun Y, Bottou L, Bengio Y, Haffner P. Gradient-based learning applied to document recognition. *Proceedings of the IEEE*. 1998;86(11):2278-2324; with permission.)

10.9% lower than the runner up. The drastic difference in performance caused a revolution within the field of AI and interest shifted back to DL. This led to many modified state-of-the-art DL networks such as the VGG network, Inception network, ResNet and others that form the cornerstones of many medical and neuroimaging applications of deep neural networks that are described in various articles elsewhere in this issue.

SUMMARY

There is a tremendous amount of interest in the potential of AI in health care. There is reason to be excited about AI and its future impact on health care, including in neuroimaging. At the same time, one must exercise caution and not fall into the trap of unrealistic expectations and hype as it pertains to AI applications. With many aspiring researchers and an expanding number of publications on DL, it is important to recognize the challenges and potential pitfalls. AI over the last few decades has repeatedly undergone moments of tremendous hype followed by the realization that some of the initial goals were out of scope. This realization causes investors to pull away from the field leading to AI winters. Projects such as IBM Watson can serve as an important example of the need for setting appropriate and realistic expectations. In 2011, after Watson gathered a lot of public attention by winning on the game show *Jeopardy!*, IBM had announced that it would begin to focus attention toward the health care field and revolutionize AI in health care in the upcoming years. Although there were several successful collaborations between hospitals and IBM, some collaborations resulted in failures.[27] Because of the high profile of the latter failures and some of the other unrealized expectations promoted both by industry and academia, there is the potential for the

public and key stakeholders to lose trust and interest, beginning a third AI winter, and overlooking and undermining the many potential important and realizable AI supported applications in health care. By providing a brief history of ML applications and AI, this article aims to provide a broader perspective on the cycles of progress in AI, in addition to many developments that preceded the current wave of innovations using DL and form the basis for many applications described in the accompanying articles in this issue. By keeping the right perspective, and understanding both the strengths and weaknesses of this important technology, one will be able to ensure the steady growth of the field without researchers and investors abandoning the field again. This could help the field of AI realize its full potential in the transformation of neuroimaging and more broadly health care.

REFERENCES

1. Devlin J, Chang M-W, Lee K, et al. BERT: pre-training of deep bidirectional transformers for language understanding. arXiv 2018. 1810.04805. Available at: https://ui.adsabs.harvard.edu/abs/2018arXiv181004805D. Accessed October 1, 2018.
2. Ren S, He K, Girshick R, et al. Faster R-CNN: towards real-time object detection with region proposal networks. Proceedings of the 28th International Conference on Neural Information Processing Systems - Volume 1; Palais des Congres de Montreal, Montreal, Canada, December 7-12, 2015.
3. Pierson HA, Gashler MS. Deep learning in robotics: a review of recent research. Adv Robot 2017;31(16): 821–35.
4. Miotto R, Wang F, Wang S, et al. Deep learning for healthcare: review, opportunities and challenges. Brief Bioinformatics 2018;19(6):1236–46.
5. McCulloch WS, Pitts W. A logical calculus of the ideas immanent in nervous activity. The Bulletin of Mathematical Biophysics 1943;5:115–33.

6. Rosenblatt F. The perceptron: a probabilistic model for information storage and organization in the brain. Psychol Rev 1958;65(6):386–408.

7. Turing AM. I.—Computing machinery and intelligence. Mind 1950;LIX(236):433–60.

8. Pinar Saygin A, Cicekli I, Akman V. Turing test: 50 years later. Minds Mach (Dordr) 2000;10(4):463–518.

9. McCorduck P. Machines who think. 2nd edition. Natick (MA): A K Peters, Ltd.; 2004.

10. Stone P, Brooks R, Brynjolfsson E, et al. Artificial intelligence and life in 2030. In: One hundred year study on artificial intelligence: report of the 2015-2016 study panel, Stanford University. Stanford (CA): Stanford University; 2016. Available at: https://ai100.sites.stanford.edu/sites/g/files/sbiybj9861/f/ai100report10032016fnl_singles.pdf. Accessed September 6, 2016.

11. Minsky M, Papert S. Perceptrons; an introduction to computational geometry. Cambridge (MA): MIT Press; 1969.

12. Lighthill J. Artificial intelligence: a general survey. London: Science Research Council; 1973.

13. Hendler J. Avoiding Another AI Winter. IEEE Intell Syst 2008;23(2):2–4.

14. McCarthy J. Some expert systems need common sense. Ann N Y Acad Sci 1984;426:129–37.

15. Rumelhart DE, Hinton GE, Williams RJ. Learning internal representations by error propagation. In: Rumelhart DE, McClelland JL, The PDP Research Group, editors. Parallel distributed processing: explorations in the microstructure of cognition, vol. 1. Cambridge (MA): MIT Press; 1985. p. 318–62.

16. Rumelhart DE, Hinton GE, Williams RJ. Learning representations by back-propagating errors. Nature 1986;323(6088):533–6.

17. Werbos P, John P. Beyond regression: new tools for prediction and analysis in the behavioral sciences. PhD thesis, Harvard University; 1974.

18. Fukushima K. Neocognitron: a self organizing neural network model for a mechanism of pattern recognition unaffected by shift in position. Biol Cybern 1980;36(4):193–202.

19. Parker DB. Learning-logic: casting the cortex of the human brain in silicon. Technical report Tr-47. Cambridge (MA): Center for Computational Research in Economics and Management Science. MIT; 1985.

20. Boser BE, Guyon IM, Vapnik VN. A training algorithm for optimal margin classifiers. Proceedings of the fifth annual workshop on Computational learning theory. Pittsburgh, PA, July 27-29, 1992.

21. Schaeffer J, Plaat A. Kasparov versus deep blue: the rematch. J Int Comput Games Assoc 1997;20:95–101.

22. Campbell M, Hoane AJ, Hsu F-h. Deep Blue. Artif Intelligence 2002;134(1):57–83.

23. Lecun Y, Bottou L, Bengio Y, et al. Gradient-based learning applied to document recognition. Proc IEEE 1998;86(11):2278–324.

24. Hinton GE, Osindero S, Teh Y-W. A fast learning algorithm for deep belief nets. Neural Comput 2006;18(7):1527–54.

25. Cireşan DC, Meier U, Gambardella LM, et al. Deep, big, simple neural nets for handwritten digit recognition. Neural Comput 2010;22(12):3207–20.

26. Krizhevsky A, Sutskever I, Hinton GE. ImageNet classification with deep convolutional neural networks. Proceedings of the 25th International Conference on Neural Information Processing Systems - Volume 1. Lake Tahoe (NV), December 3-6, 2012.

27. Strickland E. IBM Watson, heal thyself: how IBM overpromised and underdelivered on AI health care. IEEE Spectr 2019;56(4):24–31.

Knowledge Based Versus Data Based

A Historical Perspective on a Continuum of Methodologies for Medical Image Analysis

Peter Savadjiev, PhD[a,b,c,d,*], Caroline Reinhold, MD, MSc[a,d],
Diego Martin, MD, PhD[a,d], Reza Forghani, MD, PhD[a,d,e,f,g]

KEYWORDS

- Artificial intelligence • Medical image analysis • Machine learning • Computer vision
- Deep learning

KEY POINTS

- Artificial intelligence research in medical imaging has a long history.
- This review article brings a historical perspective to the evolution of artificial intelligence methods in the field of medical image analysis.
- We highlight many earlier techniques that are still highly relevant today and could be used in complement or in addition to deep learning.

INTRODUCTION

With the increasingly large amounts of digital information available in every sphere of technological activity, recent years have seen a revolution in a data-driven discovery approach to science. In the context of general image processing and analysis, deep learning methods[1] have been achieving impressive results on a large variety of tasks, for instance, in the areas of face recognition, self-driving cars, robotics and many others. These successes outside the medical world have in turn resulted in hopes for revolutionizing the computerized analysis of medical images. In fact, a perceived threat that artificial intelligence (AI) may replace radiologists within the foreseeable future has been evoked several times (for example[2]).

Nowadays, the term AI has essentially become equivalent to "deep learning" among nonspecialist circles. Part of the reason for this is the successful jump of deep learning outside research laboratories and into real-world applications. Another possible reason is the so-called Tessler theorem, or the AI effect,[3] which states that, "Intelligence is whatever machines haven't done yet." In other words, there is a tendency to reducing the definition of AI to problems that have not yet been solved. As soon as an AI-based solution to a particular task is provided, it usually stops being referred to as "AI" and becomes simply another algorithmic tool. Because of this, it is important to realize that the field of AI is in fact much broader and encompasses many techniques and tools other than deep learning.

[a] Department of Diagnostic Radiology, McGill University, Room B02 9389, 1001 Decarie Boulevard, Montreal, Quebec H4A 3J1, Canada; [b] School of Computer Science, McGill University, Montreal, Quebec, Canada; [c] Medical Physics Unit, Department of Oncology, McGill University, Montreal, Quebec, Canada; [d] Augmented Intelligence & Precision Health Laboratory (AIPHL), Department of Diagnostic Radiology, Research Institute of the McGill University Health Centre, Montreal, Quebec, Canada; [e] Segal Cancer Centre and Lady Davis Institute for Medical Research, Jewish General Hospital, Montreal, Quebec, Canada; [f] Gerald Bronfman Department of Oncology, McGill University, Montreal, Quebec, Canada; [g] Department of Otolaryngology–Head and Neck Surgery, McGill University, Montreal, Quebec, Canada
* Corresponding author. Department of Diagnostic Radiology, McGill University, Room B02 9389, 1001 Decarie Boulevard, Montreal, Quebec H4A 3J1, Canada.
E-mail address: peter.savadjiev@mcgill.ca

Neuroimag Clin N Am 30 (2020) 401–415
https://doi.org/10.1016/j.nic.2020.06.002
1052-5149/20/© 2020 Elsevier Inc. All rights reserved.

The medical image analysis algorithms that are the focus of the present review seek to achieve an automatic understanding of image content. This understanding can be focused, for example, on locating a particular organ or lesion in an image (segmentation), or on matching 2 different images of the same organs (registration). This understanding can also be broader in the sense of recovering anatomic parameters of the imaged organs, such as their shape, or in the sense of predicting the evolution of a disease based on organ/lesion appearance. We consider all such algorithms that seek to automate knowledge acquisition from images as being AI based. In doing so, we follow the traditional definition of AI, which is not limited to deep learning (which is just a subfield of machine learning), but in fact encompasses the fields of machine learning and computer vision fields in their entirety. In addition, AI includes several other fields as well, such as natural language processing and robotics, that lie outside the scope of this review. Of course, not all computer-based processing of images needs to involve AI. For instance, algorithms exist for image enhancement to assist human visualization. Image acquisition, formation, and reconstruction are also domains relying heavily on computer processing. However, for the purposes of the present review, we define medical image analysis as referring specifically to algorithms for automated knowledge acquisition from image data based on AI techniques.

In fact, automated medical image analysis has a long history that predates the mass use of deep learning. Spanning at least the last 4 decades, it has developed in tandem with advances in computer vision and machine learning, 2 of the pillars of the AI field. Many of these tools and processes are now well-understood and tend to not be considered as being AI (owing to the AI effect mentioned elsewhere in this article), at least not at the same level as current deep learning methods. Nevertheless, such methods are at the basis of many successful medical image analysis methods in wide use today. Because of that, a full understanding of AI in medical image analysis is not complete without a review of the techniques that have built the field and led it to where it currently is. Some of these techniques are mainly of historical interest, but others still play an important role today, may be complementary to deep learning, or may even outperform it in some areas.

Just like any other technique, deep learning is a tool whose performance is optimized when a specific set of constraints are met. Outside of its optimal realm of operation, however, deep learning can be surprisingly fragile and unreliable (for example[4]). For instance, it usually relies on large training sets to accurately learn the underlying patterns in the data, but this reliance often means in practice that it is the patterns associated with the majority population group that are learned the best. The performance of such systems is hampered when test data are not well-represented within the training data samples, and this is often the case in medicine with rare and/or heterogeneous diseases. To compensate for this factor, heuristic techniques such as data augmentation are typically put to use, not only to deal with the situation of class imbalance, but also to address the fact that typical medical image datasets are of much smaller size than reference nonmedical 2-dimensional image datasets, which can be in the hundreds of millions. In contrast, not only medical image datasets are much smaller, but they also consist of 2-dimensional, 3-dimensional (3D), or 4-dimensional images, each of which can be very large and contain orders of magnitude more pixels than a typical image in a common Internet training dataset such as ImageNet (http://www.image-net.org/).

To compensate for these fundamental differences in image and dataset sizes, techniques such as data augmentation and transfer learning have been put to use. In fact, they have become so indispensable that the specific way in which they are conducted oftentimes has a greater impact on the performance of a deep learning algorithm than the neural network architecture itself.[5,6] However, when dealing with a particular medical image analysis problem and when the constraints of this problem are well-understood, these generic techniques from the deep learning domain can sometimes be outperformed by alternative AI algorithms that are specifically tailored to the problem at hand (for example[7]).

The purpose of the present review article is therefore to bring to light a diversity of AI-based techniques that are well-known in the technical community of medical image analysis, but may not be as well-known to the clinical community, especially at a time when all attention is almost exclusively focused on deep learning. This review brings a historical perspective to the evolution of the field of medical image analysis, with many earlier techniques that are still highly relevant today, and could be used in complement or in addition to deep learning.

THE KNOWLEDGE-DRIVEN VERSUS DATA-DRIVEN CONTINUUM

In computer vision, but also in many other fields of science, there is a dichotomy between hypothesis-driven and data-driven methods.[8,9] In probabilistic computer vision, 2 broad classes of models exist: generative[a] and discriminative ones. Generative models ask the question, given my assumptions of how the signal was generated, what is the most likely source that generated the signal (hence the name generative)? Discriminative models, in contrast, are not interested in how the signal was generated; rather, they are only concerned with how to classify it. The most prominent example of a discriminative model in computer vision are the deep artificial neural networks known as convolutional neural networks.

Both types of approaches have benefits and drawbacks. Generative models have the advantage of allowing the incorporation of prior knowledge. Because of this, they tend to generalize well and to require much less training data than discriminative models. Their main drawback is the complexity associated with their evaluation. For a new test image, the entire signal generation model must be evaluated, which can quickly become very cumbersome, computationally expensive, and time inefficient, especially when working with a large number of images. Furthermore, in some domains, prior knowledge derived from human expertise may simply be insufficient or suboptimal in characterizing a problem.

The philosophy behind discriminative models is complementary. Instead of modeling the data generation process based on prior knowledge, they simply try to determine the aspects of the data that allow the best data categorization. In this context, the argument is often made that we should let the data tell us what is the best way to characterize images, and that it may be unnecessary to dedicate time and resources to estimating parameters of a data generation model when these parameters may, in the end, not have an influence on the final classification. Thus, by avoiding the complexity associated with a generative model, the evaluation of a discriminative model for a new test image is usually fairly straightforward, which is the main advantage of this class of models. Of course, this very same philosophy is also the source of the corresponding disadvantages. To build models with good discrimination power, large datasets are needed. Specifically, in the case of deep artificial neural network models, which can have millions of parameters, extremely large datasets are needed to appropriately train the multitude of parameters that make up the

model. As mentioned elsewhere in this article, without carefully designed mitigation strategies (which may involve the selective removal of data via undersampling), this technique introduces biases toward the majority population in the training group and greatly limits the generalization of these models in the case of data exemplars that are not part of the training distribution.[10,11] In the case of commercial face recognition software, for instance, this factor has resulted in very embarrassing gender and race biases, as recently reported.[12–14] Finally, the lack of a generative model limits the explainability of the results obtained with discriminative models, especially in the case of end-to-end deep learning, although recent advances in visualization of neural network activation maps have been able to partially mitigate this issue [for example[15]].

One of the main objectives of the present review article is to argue that it is not, in fact, necessary, to limit oneself to a dichotomy of generative versus discriminative approaches, or hypothesis-driven versus data-driven science. There is, in fact, a continuum between these 2 categories, and in this article we review examples of medical image analysis tools that fall at different points along the continuum. Furthermore, in the general computer vision community, outside of medical imaging, there has been a recent interest in combining the power of generative and discriminative models to address the limitations of each of these classes. For instance, deep generative models (not based on neural networks) have recently been proposed that take advantage of prior expert knowledge to completely outperform standard deep learning convolutional neural network models while using hundreds of times less training data and having much better generalization.[4,16,17] Applications of similar ideas in medical imaging will necessarily follow.

In this article, we provide a historical review of a sample of medical image analysis methods and locate them along the continuum between hypothesis-driven versus data-driven approaches. We will observe that, earlier on, at a time when large amounts of digital data and highly performing computers were not yet available, analysis methods tended to be naturally knowledge driven, trying to extract the maximal amount of information from a single image or a small set of images, without relying on training data. As the years

---

[a]We use the term generative here in its classical sense, not to be confused with its use in the deep learning community, where generative adversarial networks have become a popular model for synthesizing new exemplar images that look like the training images, but have been created with parameters learned with a neural network model that does not incorporate a signal generation model and/or prior knowledge.

progressed and there was an explosion both in terms of the amounts of digital data availability as well as in the availability of high-performance computing hardware, methods tended to shift toward the data-driven discovery paradigm. Today, as the best performing data-driven methods are starting to mature, we are finally coming to a point in time when we can reassess the continuum of techniques at our disposal and begin to combine in an optimal way their strengths and weaknesses to move the field forward.

THE KNOWLEDGE-DRIVEN VERSUS DATA-DRIVEN CONTINUUM: A HISTORICAL PERSPECTIVE
Fully Knowledge-Based Models

When the medical image analysis field was taking its first steps in the early 1980s, the state of the art of medical AI was embodied by so-called expert systems.[18,19] Expert systems were designed to emulate a human expert's reasoning and decision-making ability and, in those years, they were raising a debate on the role of AI in medicine,[18] reminiscent of the debate raised today by deep learning. The 2 main components of a rule-based expert system were a knowledge base, that is, a database of known facts and rules about a domain, together with a logical inference engine, whose task was to analyze the input data based on the rules and facts stored in the knowledge base. Just as with deep learning today, in those years expert systems were targeted at a very large array of domains spanning many different fields of science, engineering, and medicine. In the case of medical imaging, expert systems usually involved image processing operations (that would be considered simple by modern standards), for instance, thresholding an image and searching for geometric structures such as lines, circles, or clusters of pixels. A set of logical rules (typically in the form of IF–THEN statements) would then deduce image content based on the presence or absence of such structures (for example[20]).

These types of systems were a literal embodiment of the idea of using expert knowledge in solving a problem with AI. Given that they were based on rules entirely defined by human experts, by construction their output was fully human interpretable. However, they were riddled with many problems that ultimately led to their falling out of fashion. One problem was that maintaining the knowledge base was very cumbersome. An increasingly large number of rules were needed to capture an increasingly refined domain knowledge. However, as an increasing number of rules

were added to a knowledge base, it became increasingly difficult to ensure consistency between all of them, and to maintain an acceptable level of performance. In the end, the benefit derived from such systems did not prove of sufficient practical value in medical image analysis, especially given the limited computational resources of that era.

In parallel to expert systems for medical image analysis, the 1980s and early 1990s also saw the development of medical image analysis algorithms based on ideas borrowed from computer vision. The field of computer vision seeks to endow computers with an "understanding" of visual scenes in images. Many computer vision algorithms are inspired, at least to some extent, by biological vision. Building on the Nobel prize–winning work of Hubel and Wiesel on the neurobiology of vision,[21,22] Marr's seminal work in the 1970s postulated that vision systems are inherently hierarchical, and their objective is to create a 3D representation of the environment that can be interacted with.[23] To achieve this goal, according to Marr's philosophy, the visual system generates a hierarchy of increasingly symbolic or abstract representations of a scene, progressing from a low-level representation of localized aspects of the input image such as edges, bars, curves, and so on, to 3D models of objects. Since the early 1980s, this fundamental blueprint of vision systems has been enriched to focus not only on shape, but also on many other physical object properties such as surface reflectance, texture, motion, as well as on higher-level semantic analysis such as object recognition and categorization. However, the fundamentals of Marr's philosophy remain very much in place, and are still present in today's vision systems, even in the overall design of deep neural networks for image analysis, which are hierarchical in nature and build on low-level image descriptors to create increasingly abstract, high-level scene encodings.

To bring theory to practice, computational techniques were developed to optimize the analysis of low-level image information into higher level concepts. Knowledge-based modeling was crucial here. However, unlike expert systems, where knowledge was encoded simply as a set of rules that had to be somehow combined together, an approach that quickly reached its limits, this time knowledge was rooted in mathematical theories of optimization, physical theories of image formation and object behavior, and psychophysical findings about how the human brain processes visual information.

For instance, one of the most popular image segmentation techniques of the 1990s and early

2000s is based on the concept of active deformable models, that is, object templates (specified by expert knowledge) that deform and adapt to image content, following physics-inspired energy minimization techniques (for example[24]). The strength of this approach lies in its ability to exploit (bottom-up) constraints derived from image data, combined with (top-down, expert-driven) knowledge about the overall shape, location, size, and appearance of image structures. In addition, deformable models were among the first techniques that were able to capture the variability of biological structures over time and across individuals.

One of the simplest and most popular embodiments of a deformable model was the 'snake' model of Kass and colleagues[25] (1988). It consisted in a special type of a curve (spline) whose geometry and location are controlled by 2 energy formulations. The first is an internal energy that controls the deformations applied to the curve, by promoting continuity and smoothness and penalizing highly convoluted geometries that are not likely to represent actual object contours. The second is an external energy that controls the fitting of the curve to structures in the image. This energy is defined in terms of forces that attract the deformable model to elements of interest in the image such as edges, lines, terminations and other (user-defined) salient features. Given an initialization, the model automatically adapts itself to the image by searching for minimum energy states.

This basic model was the inspiration of many subsequent active contour/surface models for segmentation in 2-dimensional/3D images. Many of these methods were implemented with the so-called level set method, a technique originally developed in the physics literature to study the motion of propagating fronts in nature, for instance, crystal growth or flame propagation.[26] Adapted to modeling evolving fronts in image data, this framework became the basis of many medical image segmentation algorithms (for

example[27-29]). They were all built on the idea of having an evolving interface that automatically adapts to object boundaries by minimizing a combination of 2 energies: one that controls the interface's geometry by imposing geometric priors such as smoothness, and another one that attracts the evolving interface's to features of interest in the image. These features could be intensity gradients, as in earlier methods (such as[30]) or more sophisticated texture features (such as[31,32]). Representative examples of active deformable models for medical image segmentation are provided in **Figs. 1** and **2**.

The concept of balancing prior knowledge about how the world should "behave" (for instance, that object contours should be smooth), with knowledge about how the world is reflected in the data (for instance, that object contours may appear locally as edges in images) is central in computer vision and medical image analysis, and is rooted in the theory of regularization of inverse problems.[33] The smoothness prior is a very commonly used one owing to its simplicity, but a variety of more advanced geometric priors have been developed in computer vision and translated to medical image analysis. For instance, geometric constraints were developed in work by Parent and Zucker[34] for modeling curves in visual data and were then applied for white matter tractography in diffusion MR imaging data of the brain,[35] or for recovering the geometric structure of cardiac myofibers.[36] Other examples include, for instance, medial shape models (for example[37,38]).

In the 1990s, the idea of balancing internal and external forces also became a popular paradigm for registration algorithms. In this framework, external (ie, image-derived) forces driving a deformation between a source and target image were defined in terms of image similarity criteria, forcing the deformed source image to become as similar to the target image as possible. Of course, the search for the optimal mapping between 2 images based on image similarity alone is too

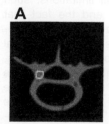
A

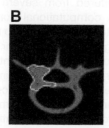
B

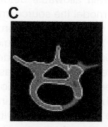
C

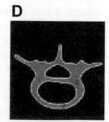
D

Fig. 1. Segmentation of a cross-sectional image of a human vertebra phantom with a topologically adaptable snake. The snake begins as a closed curve (*A*), and evolves to enclose entirely the vertebra (*D*) while changing its topology. Intermediate evolution stages are shown in (*B*) and (*C*). (*From* McInerney T, Terzopoulos D. Deformable models in medical image analysis: a survey. Med Image Anal 1(2):91-108; with permission.)

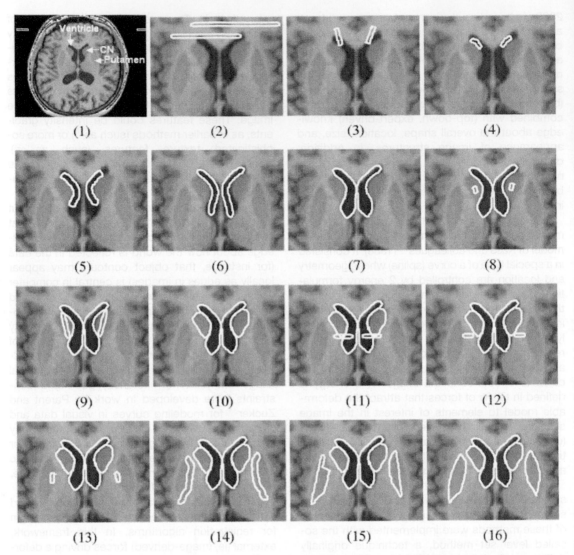

Fig. 2. Automatic brain MR image segmentation by multiple deformable models. The sequence of images illustrates the temporal progression of the segmentation process. Deformable lateral ventricle (1–7), caudate nucleus (8–10), and putamen (11–16) models are spawned in succession and progress to detect, localize, and segment the corresponding structures in the MR image. (*From* McInerney T, Hamarneh G, Shenton ME, et al. Deformable organisms for automatic medical image analysis. Med Image Anal 6(3):251-66.)

unconstrained and can easily result in unrealistic image distortions. To constrain allowable deformations, it was proposed to model the source image as embedded in a 3D deformable medium, with elastic (for example[39,40]) and/or viscous fluid (for example[41]) mechanical properties. This model defined the internal forces generated by the elasticity of the underlying material. The deformation of the source image would thus stop when the internal elasticity forces come into equilibrium with the external forces. In this framework, the equilibrium state is controlled by the Navier-Stokes equations for describing the motion of viscous fluid substances.[41]

Although conceptually attractive, this approach suffered from severe practical limitations, such as computational complexity and the fact that oftentimes tissues do not, in fact, behave according to an elastic (or viscous fluid) mechanical model. To circumvent many of these limitations, for the case of brain image registration, proposals were made for surface-based registration, where surface-based landmarks of the cortex were brought into registration first, and used as constraints to propagate a 3D deformation to register the rest of the brain volume. As a specific example, Thompson and Toga (1996)[42] proposed a method where the cortical surface is first extracted in each brain image using a deformable active surface model, in the spirit of Kass' snakes, discussed elsewhere in this article. These surfaces are then registered across individuals, using sulci, gyri, and other surface features as landmarks. This process results in a surface-based deformation field, that is, a vector field that specifies the correspondence between points on 2 individuals' brain surfaces. Finally, the full 3D volumetric warp of 1 brain image into the other is obtained by extending and interpolating the surface deformation field through the full brain volume.

Knowledge-Based Models Informed by Data Distributions

The methods discussed elsewhere in this article are representative examples of techniques that are based entirely on human knowledge used to define and constrain a solution to an image analysis problem. As such, they do not contain data-driven components. The advantage of such methods is that their results are fully interpretable and they do not require any training data, taking full advantage of the information available within a single image. However, it was quickly realized that, to fully capture population-level variability, knowledge-based modeling was not sufficient and that additional benefits can be harvested by adding statistical models of variability as measured from the data itself. Thus, the methods to be touched on this section are still based on an overall model derived from human expertise, but their parameters are now computed from a (possibly labeled) reference dataset, using probabilistic methods to determine the most likely solutions.

In the late 1990s, the field of computational anatomy rose to prominence, dedicated to studying anatomic variability in medical images. In

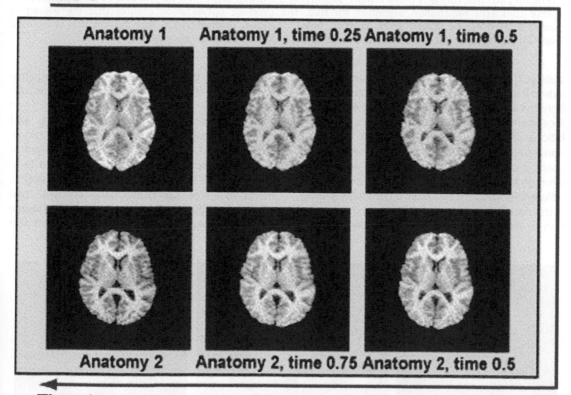

Fig. 3. In the diffeomorphic registration framework, the deformation between a source and a target image is modeled as a path in the space of diffeomorphisms (a set of mathematical image transformations). This path is parameterized with a time parameter t ranging from 0 to 1. The deformation is continuous and can be stopped at any value $0 \leq t \leq 1$ to obtain a partially deformed image. (*From* Avants B, Gee JC. Geodesic estimation for large deformation anatomical shape averaging and interpolation. Neuroimage 23(Suppl 1):S139-50; with permission.)

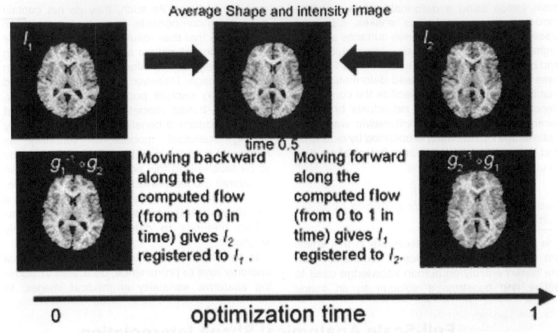

Fig. 4. The average image between 2 images can be defined as the midway point along the diffeomorphic transformation path that connects these images. Simplifying the group expression for the case of 2 images gives an inverse consistent registration algorithm for free. The geodesic optimization ensures that the averaging constraint ($E_1 = E_2$) is enforces. (*From* Avants B, Gee JC. Geodesic estimation for large deformation anatomical shape averaging and interpolation. Neuroimage 23(Suppl 1):S139-50; with permission.)

statistics, variability is defined as a measure of the extent to which data points in a distribution diverge from the average value, as well as from each other. A central question faced by researchers in computational anatomy was therefore how to define the concept of an "average image." For instance, given a population of brain images, what is the average brain? And how to define a distance (or difference) measure between a particular subject in the population and the average brain? The solution to these questions that eventually emerged

was based on the notion of diffeomorphic registration (for example[43,44]). As the name indicates, diffeomorphic registration is based on diffeomorphisms, which are differentiable and invertible transformations that preserve topology. The choice of constraining possible transformations to the space of diffeomorphisms is a form of injection of prior knowledge into the problem, which is more computationally efficient than relying on complex mechanical models. The space of diffeomorphic transformations is endowed with

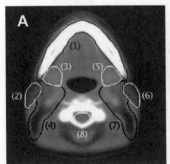
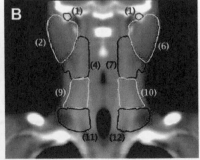
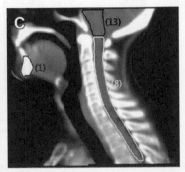

Fig. 5. Atlas built from 45 individual head and neck computed tomography images, showing the mean delineation of various anatomic structures superimposed on the atlas image, as viewed in axial (*A*), coronal (*B*) and sagittal (*C*) slices. (*From* Commonwick O, Grégoire V, Malandain G. Atlas-based delineation of lymph node levels in head and neck computed tomography images. Radiother Oncol 87(2):281-9; with permission.)

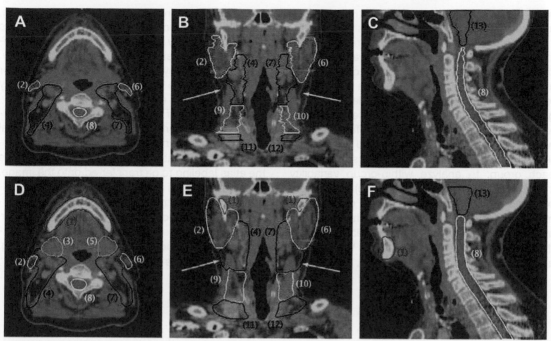

Fig. 6. Qualitative comparison of atlas-based and manual segmentations. Delineations obtained on a patient not part of the atlas construction process. (*A–C*) Manual segmentations. (*D–F*) Delineations obtained using the atlas. Structures represented: (1) mandible, (2) right parotid, (3) right submandibular gland, (4) right level II, (5) left submandibular gland. (6) left parotid, (7) left level II, (8) spinal cord, (9) right level III, (10) left level III, (11) right level IV, (12) left level IV, and (13) brainstem. (*From* Commonwick O, Grégoire V, Malandain G. (2008) Atlas-based delineation of lymph node levels in head and neck computed tomography images. Radiother Oncol 87(2):281-9; with permission.)

a metric, which allows the diffeomorphic transformation between 2 images to be described as a path in the space of diffeomorphisms. This factor allows the definition of a distance measure between 2 images as the length of this path. Furthermore, transformations can also only be carried out partially, by moving only partway along this path, as illustrated in **Fig. 3**. In this manner, the average image between 2 (or more) images can be defined as the midway point along the

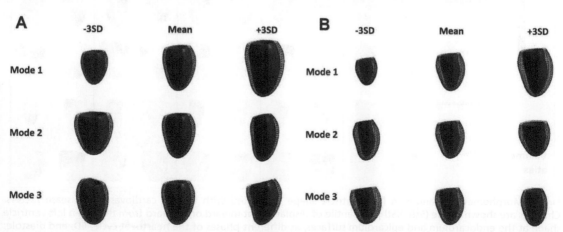

Fig. 7. Mean shape ±3 standard deviations (SD) along the first 3 principal components (modes) of shape variation at end diastole (*A*) and at end systole (*B*). (*From* Gilbert K, Bai W, Mauger C, Medrano-Gracia P, et al. Independent Left Ventricular Morphometric Atlases Show Consistent Relationships with Cardiovascular Risk Factors: A UK Biobank Study. Sci Rep. 9(1):1130; with permission.)

paths that connect these images (**Fig. 4**). This average image is often referred to as an "atlas."

In summary, the diffeomorphism framework allows for a mathematically elegant way to specify distances between images and to compute the average of a set of images, which in turns allows to compute statistical notions of variability, within groups or across groups. For instance, a common approach to study global brain differences between a healthy group and a diseased group of patients was to create an atlas representation for each group, to analyze within-group variability (more details elsewhere in this article). In addition, between-group differences can be captured by measuring differences between the 2 group atlases. Another popular use of atlases was in the detection of anomalies or lesions. When an image containing a lesion, a tumor, or another abnormality was registered with a healthy atlas, then the lesion would appear as an outlier. This is a common way of detecting and analyzing lesions in wide variety of contexts used to this day. A prominent early example is the method for detecting multiple sclerosis lesions proposed by Van Leemput and colleagues (2001).[45]

In the context of segmentation, atlases are useful not only for segmenting lesions, but also normal anatomy. When a new image is brought into registration with an atlas labeled by experts, this allows the atlas labeling to be transferred onto the image. This is the basis of many modern segmentation algorithms, one prominent example being the popular brain parcellation tool FreeSurfer (http://surfer.nmr.mgh.harvard.edu/). Atlas-based segmentation has become popular not only in brain imaging, but in other organs as well, including lung cancer[46]

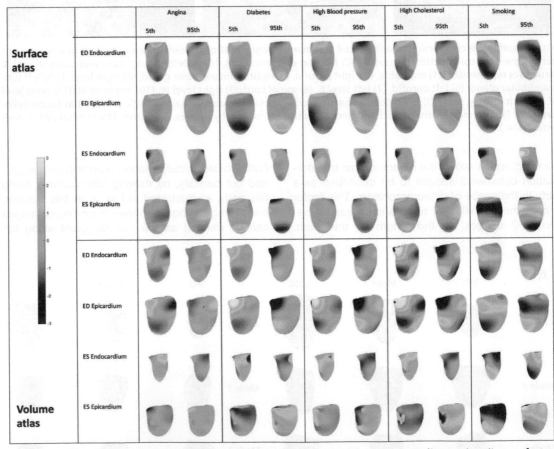

Fig. 8. Morphometric changes in left ventricle shape associated with various cardiovascular disease factors. Changes are shown as the (5th, 95th) percentile of displacement inward or outward from the mean left ventricle shape at the endocardium and epicardium surfaces, at different phases of the heartbeat cycle, ED, end diastole; ES, end systole. (*From* Gilbert K, Bai W, Mauger C, Medrano-Gracia P, Suinesiaputra A, Lee AM, Sanghvi MM, Aung N, Piechnik SK, Neubauer S, Petersen SE, Rueckert D, Young AA. (2019) Independent Left Ventricular Morphometric Atlases Show Consistent Relationships with Cardiovascular Risk Factors: A UK Biobank Study. Sci Rep. 9(1):1130.)

or head and neck computed tomography imaging.[47–50] As an example, **Fig. 5** shows an atlas computed from 45 head and neck computed tomography images. This atlas is then applied to the segmentation of a new head and neck computed tomography image (not part of the atlas construction process), with results shown in **Fig. 6** (with a comparison with manual expert segmentation).

Equipped with the notion of an average image and with a distance measure between pairs of images, it becomes then possible to treat images simply as data points in a high-dimensional space, and to apply classical statistics techniques to analyze the distribution of these data points. For instance, principal components analysis can be applied to recover the main linear modes of variation in a population. This technique was pioneered in computer vision in the late 1990s and became subsequently popular for characterizing anatomic variation in medical imaging. As recently as 2019, it was used to study the association between cardiac morphology and cardiac disease risk factors in a large cohort of the UK biobank study.[51] **Fig. 7** shows the 3 main components of shape variation for the heart's left ventricle as determined in this study. **Fig. 8** then shows the association between left ventricle shape variation and cardiac disease risk factors.

Not surprisingly, linear models for anatomic variability are not always accurate, especially in the presence of large distortions. Because of this, nonlinear methods such as manifold learning have been applied to characterize nonlinear modes of variation in a population, for instance in the study of brain development, or for characterizing various diseases (for example[52–54]).

Data-Driven Models Based on Weak Knowledge-Based Priors

Combining a knowledge-based model of image variability with parameters learned from data distributions has proven a powerful methodology, even in the presence of small datasets. For instance, Okada and colleagues (2015)[55] achieve impressive abdominal multi-organ segmentation results with only 10 to 50 training images (**Fig. 9**). With the advent of increasingly larger datasets, however, researchers started exploring the extent to which knowledge-based models can be relaxed and replaced by data-driven analysis methods.

As discussed elsewhere in this article, knowledge-based models can be complex to implement and compute, whereas data mining is relatively simple, given large enough datasets. As an example of how algorithms were developed further toward the data-driven end of the continuum, we briefly discuss sparse coding and dictionary learning. Here, models are built by learning a low-dimensional data representation, where the only prior knowledge used is a notion of sparsity, namely, that signals can be compactly

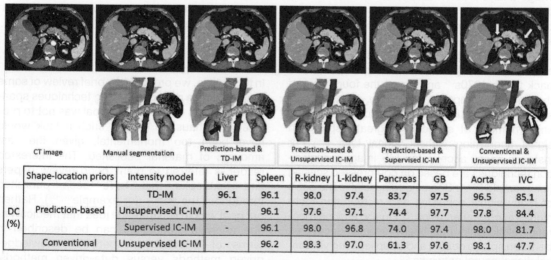

	Shape-location priors	Intensity model	Liver	Spleen	R-kidney	L-kidney	Pancreas	GB	Aorta	IVC
DC (%)	Prediction-based	TD-IM	96.1	96.1	98.0	97.4	83.7	97.5	96.5	85.1
		Unsupervised IC-IM	-	96.1	97.6	97.1	74.4	97.7	97.8	84.4
		Supervised IC-IM	-	96.1	98.0	96.8	74.0	97.4	98.0	81.7
	Conventional	Unsupervised IC-IM	-	96.2	98.3	97.0	61.3	97.6	98.1	47.7

(Column headers above data: CT image | Manual segmentation | Prediction-based & TD-IM | Prediction-based & Unsupervised IC-IM | Prediction-based & Supervised IC-IM | Conventional & Unsupervised IC-IM)

Fig. 9. Atlas based multiorgan segmentation, using 4 different datasets acquired under different imaging conditions (IC) at 2 different institutions. Dataset size ranged from 12 to 49 subjects. Different types of prior knowledge were injected into different types of intensity models (IM). Segmentation results for 1 case are shown in 2 and 3 dimensions, and Dice coefficients for individual organs are shown in a table format. CT, computed tomography; GB, gallbladder; IVC, inferior vena cava. (*From* Okada T, Linguraru MG, Hori M, Summers RM, Tomiyama N, Sato Y. (2015) Abdominal multi-organ segmentation from CT images using conditional shape-location and unsupervised intensity priors. Med Image Anal. 26(1):1-18.)

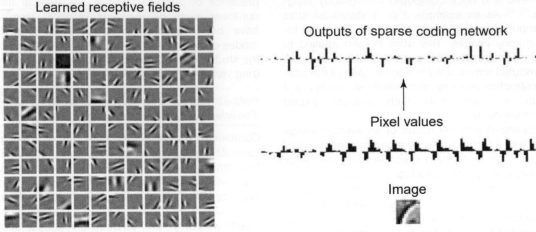

Fig. 10. (*Left*) A set of 12 × 12 pixel image patches that form a dictionary learnt by maximizing a sparse signal representation condition. Learning was performed on approximately one-half of a million image patches (of the same size) extracted from whole images of natural scenes. The dictionary patches that emerge from training are similar to visual neuronal receptive fields and are spatially localized, oriented, and bandpass (ie, selective to spatial structure at a particular scale), akin to cortical simple cells. (*Right*) An example image patch and its sparse coding via the learned dictionary. The bar chart above the image patch shows the 144 pixel values contained in the patch. These input activities are transformed into a much sparser signal representation in terms of dictionary element activation, as shown in the bar chart at the top. (*From* Olshausen BA, Field DJ (2004) Sparse coding of sensory inputs. Current Opinion in Neurobiology 14(4): 481-487; with permission.)

represented using a combination of basis functions, in a way that only a small number of basis functions is used to represent any one signal. The set of basis functions (ie, a dictionary) can be prespecified analytically, such as the sinusoids used in Fourier analysis or wavelet filters used in image analysis. Alternatively, an optimized basis can be learned for a given problem at hand, based on a training image dataset. An illustration is shown in **Fig. 10.**

The theory of sparse coding of signals in terms of a compact set of basis functions can be traced back to the 1970s[56] and lies at the foundation of the field of compressed sensing, which allows super-resolved signals to be acquired using a small number of sensors, to greatly speed up signal acquisition without signal loss.[57,58] For instance, many accelerated MR imaging acquisition techniques are based on compressed sensing (for example[59–61]). Sparse coding is also the basis of many signal denoising and restauration techniques in computer vision.[62] Finally, a close theoretic relationship has been recently uncovered between sparse coding and deep learning via convolutional neural networks.[63]

This, in a sense, completes our brief survey of the continuum between knowledge-driven versus data-driven methods in medical image analysis. We end by noting, however, that even here, at the data-driven end of this continuum, there can be found important methodologic differences

between standard deep learning techniques and other methods that may sometimes be more appropriate for a particular task. Specifically, it was recently shown that when dictionary learning was used to derive an optimized basis for digitized pathology slides, this method performed substantially better than standard transfer learning with convolutional neural networks for the classification of these images.[7]

SUMMARY

In this article, we presented a brief review of some representative medical imaging techniques spanning the last 4 decades. The goal was not to provide an exhaustive review; such a task would have been too monumental, given the vast amounts of material published. The interested reader is referred to many good review papers and textbooks that have been published throughout the years (for example[64–67]). Rather, our goal was to illustrate the idea that medical image analysis techniques can be described in terms of a continuum between knowledge-driven methods versus data-driven methods. Another objective was to emphasize the importance (and potential complementarity) of more traditional, knowledge-based AI approaches for medical image analysis to fully data-driven techniques such as deep learning. It so happened historically that knowledge-driven methods were developed first, at a time when neither large datasets nor powerful computers were available. Now that these considerations are no longer a limitation, the field's attention has heavily shifted toward data-driven analysis. As the latest and most powerful data-driven techniques are coming to maturity, and as we are becoming more aware of some of their limitations, however, it might be beneficial to revisit the full continuum of methods that are available and to study how earlier knowledge-based methods might be useful to help resolve some of the shortcomings of purely data-driven methods.

DISCLOSURE

The authors do not have any conflict of interest to report.

REFERENCES

1. LeCun Y, Bengio Y, Hinton G. Deep learning. Nature 2015;521:436–44.
2. Schier R. Artificial intelligence and the practice of radiology: an alternative view. J Am Coll Radiol 2018;15(7):1004–7.
3. Tesler L. Available at: http://www.nomodes.com/Larry_Tesler_Consulting/Adages_and_Coinages.html. Accessed March 23, 2020.
4. Yuille AL, Liu C. Deep nets: what have they ever done for vision?. 2019. Available at: https://arxiv.org/abs/1805.04025. Accessed March 23, 2020.
5. Lipton ZC, Steinhardt J. Troubling trends in machine learning scholarship. 2018. Available at: https://arxiv.org/abs/1807.03341. Accessed March 23, 2020.
6. Maier-Hein L, Eisenmann M, Reinke A, et al. Why rankings of biomedical image analysis competitions should be interpreted with care. Nat Commun 2018;9(1):5217.
7. Fischer W, Moudgalya SS, Cohn JD, et al. Sparse coding of pathology slides compared to transfer learning with deep neural networks. BMC Bioinformatics 2018;19(Suppl 18):489.
8. Kraus WL. Editorial: would you like a hypothesis with those data? Omics and the age of discovery science. Mol Endocrinol 2015;29(11):1531–4.
9. Mazzocchi F. Could Big Data be the end of theory in science? A few remarks on the epistemology of data-driven science. EMBO Rep 2015;16(10):1250–5.
10. Anand R, Mehrotra KG, Mohan CK, et al. An improved algorithm for neural network classification of imbalanced training sets. IEEE Trans Neural Netw 1993;4(6):962–9.
11. Johnson JM, Khoshgoftaar TM. Survey on deep learning with class imbalance. J Big Data 2019;6:27.

12. Buolamwini J, Gebru T. Gender shades: intersectional accuracy disparities in commercial gender classification. Proc Mach Learn Res 2018;81:1–15.
13. Buolamwini J. Gender shades: intersectional phenotypic and demographic evaluation of face datasets and gender classifiers. MIT Master's Thesis; 2017.
14. Caliskan A, Bryson JJ, Narayanan A. Semantics derived automatically from language corpora contain human-like biases. Science 2017;14:183–6.
15. Selvaraju RR, Cogswell M, Das A, et al. Grad-CAM: visual explanations from deep networks via gradient-based localization. Int J Comput Vis 2020;128:336–59.
16. George D, Lehrach W, Kansky K, et al. A generative vision model that trains with high data efficiency and breaks text-based CAPTCHAs. Science 2017;358(6368):eaag2612.
17. Kortylewski A, Liu Q, Wang H, et al. Combining compositional models and deep networks for robust object classification under occlusion. 2020. Available at: https://arxiv.org/abs/1905.11826. Accessed March 23, 2020.
18. Kinney EL. Medical expert systems. Who needs them? Chest 1987;91(1):3–4.
19. Shortliffe EH. Medical expert systems – knowledge tools for physicians. West J Med 1986;145(6):830–9.
20. Stansfield SA. ANGY: a rule-based expert system for automatic segmentation of coronary vessels from digital subtracted angiograms. IEEE Trans Pattern Anal Mach Intell 1986;2:188–99.
21. Hubel DH, Wiesel TN. Receptive fields of single neurones in the cat's striate cortex. J Physiol 1959;124(3):574–91.
22. Hubel DH, Wiesel TN. Receptive fields, binocular interaction and functional architecture in the cat's visual cortex. J Physiol 1962;160(45):106–54.
23. Marr D. Vision: a computational investigation into the human representation and processing of visual information. New York: W. H. Freeman and Company; 1982.
24. McInerney T, Terzopoulos D. Deformable models in medical image analysis: a survey. Med Image Anal 1996;1(2):91–108.
25. Kass M, Witkin A, Terzopoulos D. Snakes: active contour models. Int J Comput Vis 1988;1:321–31.
26. Osher S, Sethian JA. Fronts propagating with curvature-dependent speed: algorithms based on Hamilton–Jacobi formulations. J Comput Phys 1988;79:12–49.
27. Lorigo LM, Faugeras OD, Grimson WE, et al. CURVES: curve evolution for vessel segmentation. Med Image Anal 2001;5(3):195–206.
28. Paragios N. A level set approach for shape-driven segmentation and tracking of the left ventricle. IEEE Trans Med Imaging 2003;22(6):773–6.
29. Vasilevskiy A, Siddiqi K. Flux maximizing geometric flows. IEEE Trans Pattern Anal Mach Intell 2002;24(12):1565–78.

30. Malladi R, Sethian JA, Vemuri BC. Shape modeling with front propagation: a level set approach. IEEE Trans Pattern Anal Mach Intell 1995;17(2):158–75.

31. Chan T, Vese L. Active contours without edges. IEEE Trans Image Process 2001;10(2):266–77.

32. Paragios N, Deriche R. Geodesic active regions and level set methods for supervised texture segmentation. Int J Comput Vis 2002;46:223–47.

33. Tikhonov AN, Arsenin VY. Solution of ill-posed problems. Washington, DC: Winston & Sons; 1977.

34. Parent P, Zucker SW. Trace inference, curvature consistency, and curve detection. IEEE Trans Pattern Anal Mach Intell 1989;11(8):823–39.

35. Savadjiev P, Campbell JSW, Pike GB, et al. 3D curve inference for diffusion MRI regularization and fibre tractography. Med Image Anal 2006; 10(5):799–813.

36. Savadjiev P, Strijkers GJ, Bakermans AJ, et al. Heart wall myofibers are arranged in minimal surfaces to optimize organ function. Proc Natl Acad Sci U S A 2012;109(24):9248–53.

37. Pizer SM, Fletcher PT, Joshi S, et al. Deformable M-Reps for 3D medical image segmentation. Int J Comput Vis 2003;55(2–3):85–106.

38. Yushkevich PA, Zhang H, Gee JC. Continuous medial representation for anatomical structures. IEEE Trans Med Imaging 2006;25(12):1547–64.

39. Bajcsy R, Kovacic S. Multiresolution elastic matching. Comput Vision, Graphics, Image Process 1989;46:1–21.

40. Gee JC, Reivich M, Bajcsy R. Elastically deforming atlas to match anatomical brain images. J Comput Assist Tomogr 1993;17(2):225–36.

41. Christensen GE, Rabbitt RD, Miller MI. Deformable templates using large deformation kinematics. IEEE Trans Image Process 1996;5:1435–47.

42. Thompson P, Toga AW. A surface-based technique for warping three-dimensional images of the brain. IEEE Trans Med Imaging 1996;15(4):402–17.

43. Avants B, Gee JC. Geodesic estimation for large deformation anatomical shape averaging and interpolation. Neuroimage 2004;23(Suppl 1):S139–50.

44. Joshi S, Davis B, Jomier M, et al. Unbiased diffeomorphic atlas construction for computational anatomy. Neuroimage 2004;23(Suppl 1):S151–60.

45. Van Leemput K, Maes F, Vandermeulen D, et al. Automated segmentation of multiple sclerosis lesions by model outlier detection. IEEE Trans Med Imaging 2001;20(8):677–88.

46. Lustberg T, van Soest J, Gooding M, et al. Clinical evaluation of atlas and deep learning based automatic contouring for lung cancer. Radiother Oncol 2018;126(2):312–7.

47. Commonwick O, Grégoire V, Malandain G. Atlas-based delineation of lymph node levels in head and neck computed tomography images. Radiother Oncol 2008;87(2):281–9.

48. Fritscher KD, Peroni M, Zaffino P, et al. Automatic segmentation of head and neck CT images for radiotherapy treatment planning using multiple atlases, statistical appearance models, and geodesic active contours. Med Phys 2014;41(5):051910.

49. Lee H, Lee E, Kim N, et al. Clinical evaluation of commercial atlas-based auto-segmentation in the head and neck region. Front Oncol 2019;9:239.

50. Stapleford LJ, Lawson JD, Perkins C, et al. Evaluation of automatic atlas-based lymph node segmentation for head-and-neck cancer. Int J Radiat Oncol Biol Phys 2010;77(3):959–66.

51. Gilbert K, Bai W, Mauger C, et al. Independent left ventricular morphometric atlases show consistent relationships with cardiovascular risk factors: a UK biobank study. Sci Rep 2019;9(1):1130.

52. Aljabar P, Wolz R, Srinivasan L, et al. Combining morphological information in a manifold learning framework: application to neonatal MRI. Med Image Comput Comput Assist Interv 2010;13(Pt 3):1–8.

53. Gerber S, Tasdizen T, Joshi S, et al. On the manifold structure of the space of brain images. Med Image Comput Comput Assist Interv 2009;12(Pt 1):305–12.

54. Pless R, Souvenir R. A survey of manifold learning for images. Information Processing Society of Japan Transactions on Computer Vision and Applications 2009;1:83–94.

55. Okada T, Linguraru MG, Hori M, et al. Abdominal multi-organ segmentation from CT images using conditional shape-location and unsupervised intensity priors. Med Image Anal 2015;26(1):1–18.

56. Barlow HB. Single units and sensation: a neuron doctrine for perceptual psychology? Perception 1972;(1):371–94.

57. Candès EJ, Romberg JK, Tao T. Stable signal recovery from incomplete and inaccurate measurements. Commun Pure Appl Math 2006;59(8):1207–23.

58. Donoho DL. Compressed sensing. IEEE Trans Inf Theory 2006;52(4):1289–306.

59. Bilgic B, Setsompop K, Cohen-Adad J, et al. Accelerated diffusion spectrum imaging with compressed sensing using adaptive dictionaries. Magn Reson Med 2012;68(6):1747–54.

60. Cauley SF, Xi Y, Bilgic B, et al. Fast reconstruction for multichannel compressed sensing using a hierarchically semiseparable solver. Magn Reson Med 2015;73(3):1034–40.

61. Lustig M, Donoho D, Pauly JM. Sparse MRI: the application of compressed sensing for rapid MR imaging. Magn Reson Med 2007;58(6):1182–95.

62. Mairal J, Elad M, Sapiro G. Sparse representation for color image restoration. IEEE Trans Image Process 2008;17(1):53–69.

63. Papyan V, Romano Y, Elad M. Convolutional neural networks analyzed via convolutional sparse coding. J Mach Learn Res 2017;18:1–52.

64. Duncan J, Ayache N. Medical image analysis: progress over two decades and the challenges ahead. pattern analysis and machine intelligence. IEEE Transactions on 2000;22(1): 85–106.

65. Iglesias JE, Sabuncu MR. Multi-atlas segmentation of biomedical images: a survey. Med Image Anal 2015;24(1):205–19.

66. Zhou SK. Medical image recognition, segmentation and parsing: machine learning and multiple object approaches. San Francisco (CA): Academic Press; 2015.

67. Zhou SK, Rueckert D, Fichtinger G. Handbook of medical image computing and computer assisted intervention. San Francisco (CA): Academic Press; 2020.

Overview of Machine Learning: Part 2
Deep Learning for Medical Image Analysis

William Trung Le, BSc[a,b,1], Farhad Maleki, PhD[c,1],
Francisco Perdigón Romero, MSc[a], Reza Forghani, MD, PhD[c,d,e,f],
Samuel Kadoury, PhD[a,b,*]

KEYWORDS

• Deep learning • Medical imaging • Health care • Convolutional neural network • Image registration
• Image synthesis • Treatment planning • Radiology

KEY POINTS

• Radiological imaging data for H&N contains a wealth of information suitable for feature extraction using deep learning methods to characterize various pathologies.
• Convolutional neural networks (CNN) have recently become highly effective in multiple medical imaging tasks including anatomical classification, segmentation and registration, as well as disease progress prediction, and image reconstruction.
• Various experimental and ethical considerations still need to be addressed to ensure successful deployment of deep learning models in clinical settings.

INTRODUCTION

Innovations in deep learning continue to result in breakthroughs across multiple fields, including computer games,[1,2] autonomous driving,[3] predictive health care,[4,5] and natural language processing.[6,7] These breakthroughs can be attributed to improvements in graphical processing units technology allowing faster model training[8]; the emergence of accessible development frameworks such as TensorFlow,[9] Keras,[10] PyTorch,[11] MXNet,[12] and Caffe[13]; and the increasing volume of data available for model training.[14] Artificial neural networks (ANN) were originally modeled after the biological neurons and their synaptic connections in the brain and can be considered the building blocks for deep learning architectures.[15–17] With ANNs, the flow of synaptic pulses can be seen as a hierarchical feature extractor.[8] As information is propagated through the layers of neurons, the internal representation captures increasingly more abstract and complex relationships. This is the motivation for the development of "deep" networks, with many layers for processing large and complex data.

Preprint submitted to *Neuroimaging Clinics* February 27, 2020.
Funding Information: Dr Samuel Kadoury is a Canada Research Chair (CRC) in Medical Imaging and Assisted Intervention.
^a Polytechnique Montreal, PO Box 6079, succ. Centre-ville, Montreal, Quebec H3C 3A7, Canada; ^b CHUM Research Center, 900 St Denis Street, Montreal, Quebec H2X 0A9, Canada; ^c Augmented Intelligence & Precision Health Laboratory (AIPHL), Department of Radiology and Research Institute of the McGill University Health Centre, 1001 Decarie Boulevard, Montreal, Quebec H4A 3J1, Canada; ^d Segal Cancer Centre, Lady Davis Institute for Medical Research, Jewish General Hospital, 3755 Cote Ste-Catherine Road, Montreal, Quebec H3T 1E2, Canada; ^e Gerald Bronfman Department of Oncology, McGill University, Montreal, Quebec, Canada; ^f Department of Otolaryngology - Head and Neck Surgery, McGill University, Montreal, Quebec, Canada
¹ Co-first author.
* Corresponding author.
E-mail address: samuel.kadoury@polymtl.ca

This was shown in 2012 during the ImageNet Large-Scale Visual Recognition Challenge,[18] previously dominated by classic computer vision methods. The AlexNet model used a deep convolutional neural network (CNN), leading to a substantial reduction in error rate compared with the classic computer vision methods.[19] This success revolutionized image processing research and applications.

In medical imaging, computed tomography (CT), MR imaging, and ultrasound images are prevalent. These imaging modalities can be used for diagnosis, treatment planning, disease monitoring, and evaluation of response to therapy. Traditionally, radiologists perform these analyses, relying on human-discernible visual features. However, this manual approach requires years of specialized training, and the inherent complexity of these types of images can make certain manual tasks and the subjective process laborious, time-consuming, and prone to interobserver variability. Furthermore, increasing evidence suggests that the complex quantitative information on medical images is underutilized using current approaches. Deep learning thus offers multiple benefits compared with previous techniques: the ability to perform medical image analysis for identification of high-order complex features, performing different classification tasks or predictive modeling, and accelerating image processing tasks. These advantages will facilitate deployment in the clinical workflow. This article provides the fundamental background required to understand and develop deep learning models used for medical image processing. The authors cover the main deep learning architectures such as feedforward and recurrent neural networks and their variants and also provide use cases of such applications in medical image processing.

DEEP LEARNING ARCHITECTURES
Feedforward Neural Networks

In a feedforward network, the information flow between computational units in the network can be represented as a directed acyclic graph, where the information flows from the inputs to outputs. In other words, there is no path in which the output of a computational unit is fed back into itself. Typical examples of feedforward networks include multilayer perceptrons (MLPs), convolutional neural networks, autoencoders, and generative adversarial networks (GANs).

Multilayer Perceptrons

MLPs are the quintessential feedforward networks. The term is sometimes used

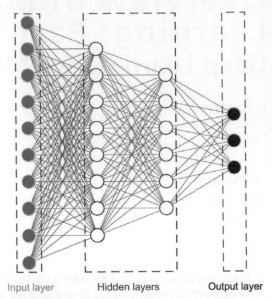

Fig. 1. A multilayer perceptron. Each artificial neuron is represented by a circle in white or blue color. The network consists of an input layer (in *green*), an output layer (in *blue*), and 2 hidden layers (in *white*). Each edge represents a weight for the network. These weights define the network and are determined through a training process.

interchangeably with feedforward networks. An MLP, as depicted in **Fig. 1**, consists of several layers, each with one or more artificial neurons. Each neuron accepts one or more inputs. First, each input is multiplied by a weight. Then the summation of all weighted inputs and a bias value are calculated. Next, an activation function is applied to the summation, and the output of the activation function is considered as the neuron's output. The outputs of the neurons from each layer are used as inputs for the neurons in the next layer of the network.

Network weights, often referred to as network parameters, define the output of the network for a given input. These weights are often initialized randomly. Then during an iterative process, referred to as the training process (see Section 3), the optimal weight assignment for the network is sought. During the training process, a loss function is used to measure the optimality of a given weight assignment for the network.

Activation functions are used to introduce nonlinearity to the network and make it possible for the network to learn complex nonlinear functions. Rectified linear unit (ReLU) and its variants, Sigmoid, and Tanh are commonly used in neural networks.[8,20,21] ReLU and its variants are commonly used for neurons in hidden layers. Sigmoid is commonly used in the output layers of

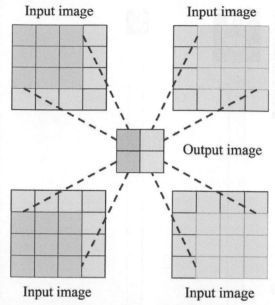

Fig. 2. A 3 × 3 convolution. A convolution slides over the input and generates an output. This allows the same local feature to be extracted anywhere within the input, which means fewer parameters to be learned.

networks designed for classification. In multiclass classification, softmax function (also known as softargmax) is applied to the output of the network to generate a class probability distribution.

Convolutional neural networks

Training MLP for tasks with a large number of inputs requires a substantial amount of training examples that might not always be available. For example, using a 1000 by 1000 grayscale image (width: 1000 and height: 1000) leads to an input dimension of 1,000,000. Building an MLP for processing such images is impractical. In addition, there are high spatial dependencies between neighboring pixels in an image. CNNs use these spatial dependencies and build on MLPs by replacing neurons with convolutions (**Fig. 2**) and pooling operators.[8] These operators are applied to a neighborhood rather than the whole input. This approach has 2 primary advantages: sparse connectivity and parameter sharing.[8] Using convolutional kernels reduces the number of parameters compared with using fully connected layers in MLPs. This reduces the memory requirements and makes it possible to achieve a better performance. Also, the kernel is repeatedly applied to each region of the image: this allows its parameters to be shared across the image. This is in contrast to MLPs where a weight is only associated with an input from the previous layer.

A convolution operator—also referred to as a convolutional kernel or filter—computes a weighted linear combination of its parameters and the corresponding inputs from the region where the filter is applied.

A CNN consists of several convolution or pooling layers (**Fig. 3**). Each convolution layer includes several kernels. The output of each layer can then be used as the input for the next layer. Because convolutions act as local feature extractors, pooling operations are necessary to allow global feature combinations. A pooling operation summarizes the corresponding inputs from the region where the operator is applied. For example, the output of a max-pooling operator is the maximum of the corresponding values where the operator is applied, and this can be used to reduce the dimensions of the intermediate representations. Pooling operators can reduce the memory requirement and the sensitivity to small translations in the input, as well as increase the effective receptive field for future convolution operators.

Autoencoders

Autoencoders are a family of feedforward networks commonly used for providing a low-dimensional representation of data.[8] An advantage of autoencoders is that they can be trained in an unsupervised manner without labeled data. An autoencoder has 2 components: an encoder and a decoder. For a given input x, the encoder tries to provide a low-dimensional representation y from x. The decoder, on the other hand, tries to reconstruct the input x using y, that is, the low-dimensional representation generated by the encoder. The intuition behind autoencoders is that if y is an accurate representation of x, it should hold enough information to reconstruct x.

The autoencoder can be trained end-to-end using the backpropagation algorithm (see Section 3). **Fig. 4** illustrates a typical autoencoder, which is also referred to as an undercomplete autoencoder. Several other variants of autoencoders exist: contractive autoencoders,[22,23] denoising autoencoders,[24] and variational autoencoders.[25]

Sensitivity to small variations and noise in the training data is one of the challenges an autoencoder might encounter. To address this challenge, contractive autoencoders add a specific component to the loss function to penalize network weights that lead to sensitivity to small variation in the data. In mathematical terms, this component corresponds to the Frobenius norm of the Jacobian matrix of the activations in the encoder. In denoising autoencoders, a different approach is used to address these challenges. During the training process, inputs are corrupted by

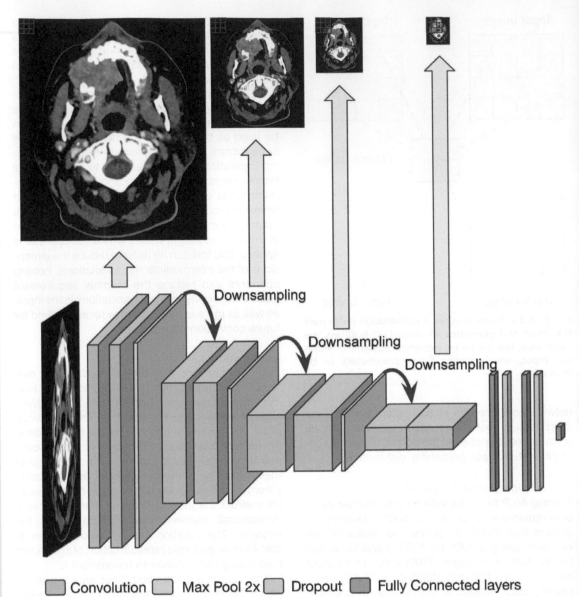

Downsampling

Downsampling

Downsampling

⬜ Convolution ⬜ Max Pool 2x ⬜ Dropout ⬛ Fully Connected layers

Fig. 3. A CNN-based network for image classification. Successive convolution and downsampling through max pooling reduce the input size while increasing the kernel's receptive field. The original images at the top were used to represent the increase in the receptive field while being a reference for the dimensionality reduction of the intermediate representations as the result of applying max pooling. For an image classification task, the CNN component is followed by an MLP to convert the deep features generated by CNN to a class probability distribution.

introducing small random noises. Then the network is trained to learn the actual input before the corruption. Corrupted inputs can be made through a stochastic process such as adding Gaussian noise or masking noise.[26]

Generative adversarial networks
GANs are composed of 2 networks: a generator and a discriminator, as shown in **Fig. 5**.[27] These

networks are trained in parallel with opposite goals. The generator synthesizes data from scratch, often using random inputs. The discriminator on the other hand receives either a ground truth from the target domain or a synthetic output, which is produced by the generator, and tries to distinguish the true outputs from the synthetic ones.

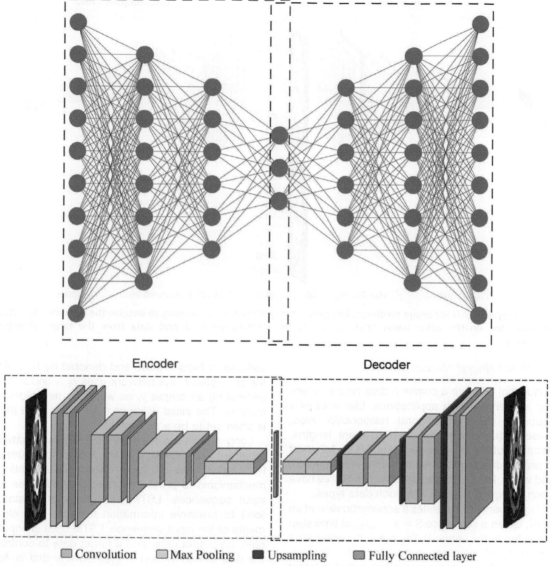

Encoder   Decoder

☐ Convolution   ☐ Max Pooling   ■ Upsampling   ☐ Fully Connected layer

Fig. 4. Typical autoencoders based on MLP (*top*) and CNN (*bottom*). The network consists of 2 components: the encoder and the decoder. The encoder, represented within the red box, transforms the input to a lower dimensional space. For the MLP-based autoencoder, the low-dimensional representation is the output of the 3 neurons (*green*). For the CNN-based autoencoder the representation is the output of the convolution layer (*green*). The decoder's task is to reconstruct the input using the low-dimensional representations generated by the encoder.

During the training process, generators incorporate feedback from the discriminator to improve its performance, where the performance is measured based on the percentage of synthesized data classified by the discriminator as being from the target domain. Training a GAN model is a balancing act between the generator and the discriminator performance. An overperformance by either side leads to an overfitting situation where the synthesized output becomes meaningless. Convergence thus occurs when a Nash equilibrium is attained: real and synthetic data become indistinguishable.

In medical imaging, GANs are often used for image registration[28–30] or image synthesis tasks.[31–35] In registration tasks, the generator outputs a transformation, and the discriminator must distinguish the warped image from the alignment target image. Synthesis tasks often revolve around generating a new synthetic view of the input image, such as MR imaging to CT synthesis[35] or generation of 3-dimensional (3D) organ volumes from 2D single-slice scans.[36,37] GAN may also be used for data augmentation, as discussed in Section 3 (see **Fig. 5**).

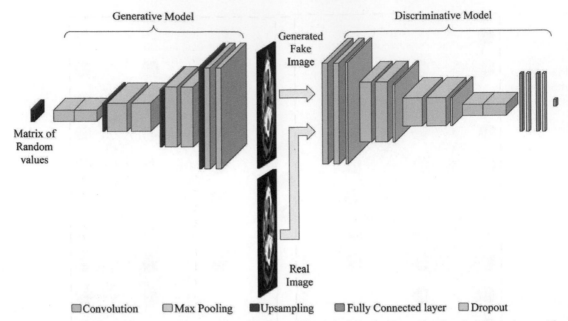

| Convolution | Max Pooling | Upsampling | Fully Connected layer | Dropout |

Fig. 5. A typical GAN for image synthesis. The generator synthesizes data aiming to deceive the discriminator. The discriminator, on the other hand, tries to classify the synthesized data and data from the target domain accurately.

Recurrent Neural Networks

Sequential data are a common data type in scientific and engineering applications. Elements of a sequence have a temporal relationship. Also, these sequences might have different lengths. Because of these characteristics, MLPs fall short in processing sequential data such as text, audio, and video. Recurrent neural networks (RNNs) have been designed to work with such data types.

Fig. 6 (panel A) illustrates a schematic view of an RNN. Given a sequence $S = x_1,...,x_n$, at time step t, x_t is fed to the network. The network preserves a summary of previous data elements, that is, $x_1,...,x_{t-1}$. This summary is often called a latent variable or hidden state and denoted by h_{t-1}. At the time step t, the network uses h_{t-1} and x_t for generating an output y_t as well as a new hidden state h_t. The initial value of the hidden state (h_0) is often set to be a zero vector.

Long short-term memory (LSTM)[38] and gated recurrent units (GRU)[39,40] are 2 commonly used RNN architectures. These architectures use gating mechanisms to preserve longer dependencies in input sequences. LSTM uses an internal state (cell) to preserve information from the key elements of the input sequence. LSTM uses an input gate, an output gate, and a forget gate to control the flow of information in the network, that is, to update the cell and hidden states. GRU is a

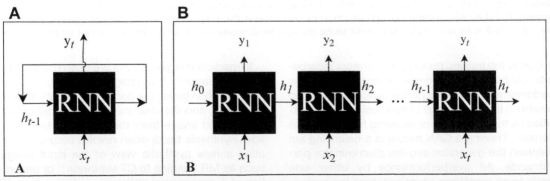

Fig. 6. A schematic view of a typical RNN. The RNN has been visualized as a black box. At each time step t, the RNN accepts a hidden state (h_{t-1}) from the previous time steps ($x_1,...,x_{t-1}$) as well as an input. The RNN then generates an output (y_t) and a new hidden state (h_t). Panel B shows the computational logic of the same network. The initial hidden state (h_0) is often set to be a zero vector.

variation of LSTM. It is a simpler architecture with no cell and with only reset and update gates. GRU has less parameters due to its lack of output gate and may achieve higher performance when working with small datasets.[40] In general, LSTMs have more capacity and are more powerful in comparison to GRUs.[41]

TRAINING AND VALIDATION OF DEEP LEARNING MODELS
Training Deep Learning Models

After data acquisition and network architecture design/selection, the network should be trained to determine the weights that lead to an optimal or near-optimal solution for the task at hand. First, network weights are initialized through a stochastic process. Xavier initialization[42] and Kaiming initialization[43] are some commonly used network initialization methods. The training of deep learning networks is carried out through an optimization process, where the objective is to minimize the error obtained through a cost function. This function—also referred to as loss function—represents the difference between the network outputs from the desired outputs. To correct the error, the backpropagation algorithm is used to modify network weights depending on their contribution to the calculated loss. This process is repeated several times until a stopping criterion is achieved.[17]

The loss function may vary depending on the task at hand. For regression tasks, where the model outputs are continuous values, the most commonly used loss functions are mean squared error and mean absolute error, also referred to as L1 loss. For classification tasks, where the model output is a categorical variable, the most common loss functions are cross-entropy and hinge loss. For segmentation tasks, the most commonly used loss functions are pixel accuracy, intersection over union—also referred to as Jaccard Index—and Dice coefficient.

Backpropagation

The learning process for a neural network consists of 2 phases: a stimulus presentation phase followed by a model adaptation phase. In the first step, an input is fed to and processed by the network, resulting in a prediction output that is compared with the expected output using a loss function. This difference, also called the error or loss value, can then be used to numerically update the parameters (weights and biases) of the network in order to minimize the loss value. The backpropagation algorithm calculates the gradient of the loss function with respect to network parameters through the chain rule, which is a mathematical formula for calculating the derivatives of a composite function in an efficient way. After calculating the gradients, the network parameters can then be updated incrementally to minimize the future loss with the given input.[8]

Considerations for Training Deep Learning Models

Bias versus variance
Differentiating training error, generalization error, and Bayes error are crucial for developing and deploying deep learning models successfully. Training error refers to the error made by a model when applied to the data used during model training. Generalization error, on the other hand, is the error made by a model when applied to previously unseen data. These data must not be used for the training or fine-tuning steps nor as well as for the design or selection of the model architecture. Finally, the Bayes error—also known as irreducible error—is the lowest achievable error for a task using a given dataset. Most often it is not possible to mathematically calculate Bayes error. Therefore, an estimate for it is used: for example, the predictions made by a council of experts can be used for estimating Bayes error. It should be noted that unlike training and generalization errors, Bayes error is independent of a given model; rather, it is defined for a task based on a given dataset. Simply put, Bayes error is an indicator of the best possible algorithm performance for a task given a specific dataset.

When developing deep learning models, the available data are often divided into 3 subsets: training, validation, and test data. Training data are used to train the model through an optimization process. Test data are used to estimate the generalization error for the trained model. Validation data are used to tune model hyperparameters, for example, number of layers in an MLP, and also to avoid overfitting to the training data.

Overfitting and underfitting are 2 fundamental concepts in machine learning. Overfitting happens when a model achieves a small training error but relatively large generalization error, that is, there is a falsely optimistic performance of the model. Underfitting, on the other hand, happens when a model achieves a large training error relative to the Bayes error.

Overfitting and underfitting can also be explained by the bias-variance trade-off. Bias error refers to the error made due to erroneous or oversimplifying assumptions made when building a model. Errors due to a high variance happen when the model becomes too sensitive to small fluctuations or noise in the training data. Thus, a model with high bias leads to underfitting, whereas a model with high variance leads to overfitting. Using linear regression to model a highly nonlinear relationship between dependent and independent variables leads to high bias error and such a model will underfit. On the other hand, using a deep MLP for capturing a linear relationship leads to high variance error and such a model will overfit. Therefore, finding a bias-variance trade-off is essential in machine learning applications.

Among common approaches to deal with overfitting are using larger training datasets and controlling model complexity through the proper use of regularization, dropout,[44] and early stopping.[8] Also, changing network architecture is used to achieve a trade-off between bias and variance. Underfitting usually happens due to insufficient training or model capacity. A more detailed discussion of machine learning algorithm validation is provided in a separate review article in this issue.

Data augmentation
One approach to deal with overfitting is to use large-scale datasets for training deep learning models. However, this is often not an option in the biomedical domain, as it requires resources that might not be accessible in a timely and cost-effective way; because of legal, ethical, or privacy considerations; or because the disease being studied is rare or the biological process of interest (eg, a complex molecular profile) may only be available on a small set of patients. Data augmentation refers to computational methods used to generate new samples from existing ones. These new samples, together with the original samples, can then be used for training a machine learning model. These methods have been extensively used in image processing tasks.[45] Image augmentation methods include simple transformations such as cropping, affine transformations, color space transformation, random erasing, noise injection, elastic deformation,[46] as well as more complex approaches such as GAN-based data augmentation methods.[32]

Data imbalance
A common challenge when working with medical data is data imbalance, also known as class imbalance. This imbalance happens when a disproportionate ratio of observations exists in each class or observation category. For a dataset, the class imbalance is measured using the imbalance ratio defined as the ratio of the number of observations in the majority class to that of the minority class. The majority and minority classes are defined to be the classes with the largest and smallest number of observations, respectively.

Class imbalance, if not addressed properly, might hamper developing generalizable models. Many methods for addressing class imbalance exist.[47] Oversampling, undersampling, and data augmentation are 3 common approaches for addressing data imbalance. These techniques attempt to generate a new balanced dataset from the original imbalanced one. Oversampling introduces extra samples into classes with a smaller number of observations. For each class, these additional samples are generated through resampling with replacement from the members of the class itself. In undersampling, on the other hand, samples from classes with a larger number of observations are discarded to reduce the imbalance. A shortcoming of these resampling techniques is that they change the data distribution, and the model trained with the resampled data might not achieve the optimal results. In addition, undersampling might lead to overfitting for datasets with high imbalance ratios. Data augmentation can also be used to introduce more samples to the class(es) with a smaller number of samples. Another method for dealing with data imbalance is defining a loss function to be in favor of classes with a small number of observations, that is, to impose larger penalties for the error made using samples from small classes when training the model.

Transfer learning
Transfer learning refers to using knowledge gained from a source domain to solve problems in a target domain that is related to, but not the same as, the source domain. Because of the resource-intensive nature of deep learning, transfer learning has been widely used.[5,48–51]

In the presence of large public datasets, such as ImageNet,[18] an initial model is trained on these datasets. Then the pretrained model is fine-tuned on a target domain, where the required resources for training the model from scratch might not be available. A large number of pretrained models exist for image processing tasks. Therefore, transfer learning has been widely used for medical image analysis, where acquiring large datasets is often impractical.

For classification tasks, the number of classes in the target domain might differ from that of the pretrained model. Therefore, the classifier component of the pretrained model is replaced with a new classifier that suits the target domain. This new resulting model is then trained using the available data from the target domain.

Deep Learning for Medical Imaging

Medical imaging with a broad range of domains, modalities, and tasks is a field rich in potential for deep learning applications. In this section, the authors provide use cases of applications of deep learning in medical imaging.

Classification

Classification is a process through which the category of each observation must be predicted among a set of predetermined categories. Detecting the presence of a disease, classifying a lesion, and predicting the response to a line of treatment are examples of classification tasks conducted using medical imaging. The resulting models can provide added diagnostic or prognostic benefits in a noninvasive manner. In this section, the authors cover some classification use cases in medical imaging.

- To predict transarterial chemoembolization response level in hepatocellular carcinoma, Peng and colleagues[49] used a ResNet model[52] pretrained on the ImageNet dataset[18] and fine-tuned on their internally collected 789 patients' CTs and achieved 85.1% and 82.8% prediction accuracies.
- For tracking disability progression of patients with multiple sclerosis after 1 year, Tousignant and colleagues[50] proposed a CNN approach based on an Inception model[53] trained on a proprietary brain MR imaging dataset with 5 different sequences as inputs. They achieved a 66.0% receiver operating characteristic area under the curve (AUC) score, which was improved to 70.1% with the introduction of 2 extra lesion mask sequences as input images.
- Using transfer learning, Zhou and colleagues[51] built 3 different binary classifiers for distinguishing benign and malignant tumors from CT images. Their first model, which was called the image-level model, was built based on an Inception model[53] adopted for binary classification of CT slices. In their second and third models, which were called patient-level models, they first extracted a feature vector for each slice of the CT. These features were extracted from a trained version of the image-level model. The second model concatenated these feature vectors and fed them into a max pooling layer, followed by a shallow MLP-based binary classifier. The third model used a GRU-based binary classifier that accepted these feature vectors as sequential inputs. They reported that the patient-level models

achieve better results compared with the image-level models.

- To predict breast cancer risk from mammograms, McKinney and colleagues[5] developed an ensemble of 3 deep learning systems, namely lesion model, breast model, and case model. The average of the predicted risk scores was then used as the ensemble prediction. For each patient, they used craniocaudal and mediolateral oblique views of the left and right breasts. In the lesion model, they used RetinaNet[54] to detect regions of interest (ROIs) and their corresponding confidence scores. Then 10 ROIs with the highest confidence score as well as their corresponding regions from contralateral breast were selected. Each ROI and its corresponding region were fed to a MobileNetV2[55] to predict a cancer risk score. Ten calculated risk scores were then combined to calculate a case-level score. The Breast model used a ResNet[56] module as the feature extractor. Then per breast features were fed to another residual network[52] to make the case-level prediction. Case model also used a ResNet feature extractor.[52] The extracted features for each view of the left and right breast were concatenated and fed to an MLP for making the case-level predictions. They trained and evaluated the model using 2 large datasets and reported reductions in false-positive rates of 9.4% and 2.7% and reduction in false-negative rates of 5.7% and 1.2% for these datasets compared with predictions made by experts.

Segmentation

In semantic segmentation, the goal is to delineate the boundaries of anatomic or pathologic structures of interest. The results are used to guide treatment target planning, to aid multimodal image registration, or to aid operative navigation systems. U-Net[57] and its variants have been widely used for segmentation in the medical imaging field. **Fig. 7** illustrates U-Net architecture.

- Hashemi and colleagues[58] developed a 3D fully convolutional architecture based on DenseNet blocks and an asymmetric loss for infant brain MR imaging white matter, gray matter, and cerebrospinal fluid segmentation. By having the model learn 2 of the 3 labels in parallel and taking the complement to generate the contours for the third (gray matter), they achieved a 96% Dice score.
- Sun and colleagues[59] demonstrated that hippocampus segmentation can be improved by using a V-Net[60] coupled with an auxiliary loss

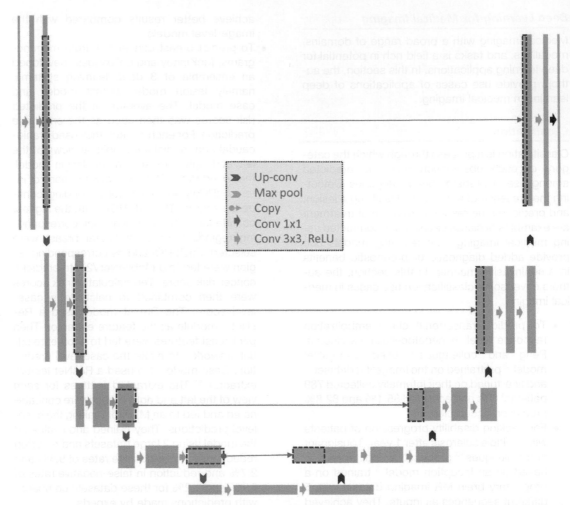

⮞	Up-conv
⮞	Max pool
↔	Copy
⬇	Conv 1x1
⬆	Conv 3x3, ReLU

Fig. 7. U-Net architecture[57] is made of a contracting path followed by an expansive path. In the contracting path, a sequence of convolution and pooling operators produces a dense representation of the input image. In the expansive path, a sequence of convolution and upsampling operators is used to generate the segmentation mask. To be able to use both high-level and low-level features, U-Net used a crop and copy operator.

for brain state classification. Hippocampal size is a useful feature for monitoring Alzheimer disease progression. They showed that taking the embedded representation of the network and the output mask as input to a classification subnetwork as an additional constraint, segmentation results improved to 91.6% Dice score.

- Yin and colleagues[61] developed a novel method to segment kidney ultrasound images using a combination of 2 deep learning models. The first model computes an organ boundary distance map using a pretrained version of VGG model[62] feature extractor modified with atrous convolutions.[63] This distance map has the advantage of reducing the pixel-wise organ to background class

imbalance. The predicted kidney boundary map was then fed to a pretrained DeepLab[64] segmentation network. Yin and colleagues reported a 93% Dice score on their privately acquired dataset.

Registration

Image registration is the task of aligning 2 images together. Image registration is required when a one-to-one mapping between 2 acquired images is not possible by simply overlaying one image on the other. This is the case when these images are from different scan times, causing a shift in the anatomic structures due to movement. These misalignments might imply different visual features of the same area. In this section, the authors provide examples of deep learning applications for image registration.

- de Vos and colleagues[65] introduced an unsupervised method that takes a pair of images through a CNN and outputs affine or B-spline deformation parameters. It shows comparable performance to conventional methods for cardiac cine MR imaging and chest CT registration while being substantially faster to compute.
- Balakrishnan and colleagues[66] introduced the VoxelMorph method, which instead outputs a deformation field via a U-Net model, outperforming the state-of-the-art results on brain MR imaging registration tasks.
- Shen and colleagues[67] developed a 2-step ensemble model combining both the affine and the deformable transformations. Their U-Net generated a velocity field, from which a deformation field was computed. This has the advantage of ensuring better fluid mechanics properties and smoother deformations.
- Eppenhof and colleagues[68] devised a method to train the U-Net–based model on pulmonary CT by starting with lower resolution images and progressively increasing them. To do so, they restricted the depth of their model and increased it over time, which allows the model to learn coarse-to-fine grained deformations.

Reconstruction, Synthesis, and Denoising

In certain medical applications, converting images between different modalities might be necessary due to better resolution, contrast to visualize clinically relevant details, or reducing radiation doses. Therefore, a model should synthesize an instance of anatomic structures in the target modality using another modality as input. Paired multimodal datasets are often rare in the medical domain; this makes GANs a well-suited option for such image synthesis tasks.

- Yang and colleagues[69] used a CycleGAN[70] to synthesize CT from MR for patients with brain tumor. This method consists of enforcing the model to be able to generate modalities from either direction. In their qualitative evaluation, experts could not distinguish the real from the synthesized pairs.
- Rubin and Abulnaga[71] developed a CT to MR model based on conditional GANs, a variant where both the generator and discriminator also accept a source domain image as input. They showed that the

resulting MR imaging yielded improvements in their pipeline to improve stroke lesion segmentation.
- Bass and colleagues[72] developed a novel variant of the conditional GAN with added capsule blocks[73,74] for cortical axons microscope images. They showed that the resulting images were realistic enough to be used to train a segmentation pipeline that tested successfully on real datasets.

In the medical imaging field, reconstruction refers to transforming images from a physical domain—eg, intensity variations of the electromagnetic field for MR imaging—to images that humans can understand. Generally, these reconstruction processes are computationally expensive and difficult to parallelize. Deep learning has been used to learn and enhance such transformations.[75,76] Examples include accelerating the use of deep learning to enable acceleration of acquisition of an MR imaging sequence while preserving diagnostic information or the use of deep learning for denoising medical images.[77,78] Often noisy images prevent the correct diagnosis; therefore, denoising can add a substantial value to diagnosis and treatment workflow. To achieve such a task, a model must receive an image as input and generate a denoised version of the image as the output. Therefore, fully convolutional autoencoders have been used for such a task.[77,78]

LIMITATIONS AND FUTURE DIRECTIONS

Unlike traditional machine learning models, where the performance plateaus at some point and using more data does not improve the model performance leading to an underfitting situation, the performance of deep learning models improves as the number of training examples increases. Therefore, data availability is essential for developing deep learning models. Data availability can pose a problem in the medical imaging field where training data are scarce due to the lack of infrastructure, expert annotations, or patient privacy concerns or simply due to the rarity of the phenotype/disease under study.

Transfer learning techniques have been considered to alleviate the scarcity of training data. Using large pretrained models to extract latent features has proved to be successful in many medical imaging tasks.[5,48–51] These pretrained models are trained on public datasets from domains different from the medical domain. For example, many available pretrained models have been trained on the ImageNet dataset, which is a collection of ordinary pictures. Therefore, the extracted features from these pretrained models could potentially be improved if the pretrained models were instead trained on medical image datasets. Medical images often have different visual characteristics and a higher resolution and pixel intensity depth. Considering the availability of many small- and medium-sized public dataset of medical images—eg, datasets from the Grand Challenge in Medical Imaging and the Cancer Imaging Archive—a data aggregation attempt for building a large-scale medical imaging dataset and providing pretrained models based on this dataset may benefit the research community and facilitate the deployment of methods built on these domain-specific pretrained models in clinical setting.

Medical images come in a variety of modalities such as radiographs, ultrasound, CT, MR imaging, PET, and other nuclear medicine scans, to mention the most common ones. One may also consider digital histopathology slides as medical images. These modalities have different spatial and depth resolution. Also, using different modality-specific acquisition parameters—T1 versus T2 weighting of MR imaging scans or adding a contrast agent—provides trade-off for visibility of certain substructures. Finally, medical images are also affected by device- or manufacturer-specific differences, varying reconstruction parameters that can vary between institutions and even within the same institution, and different maneuvers or positioning that may be used for targeted evaluation depending on the specific body part. These factors pose a new dimension of complexity on top of the complex nature of regular image processing tasks. Most of the deep learning models in the literature often demonstrated state-of-the-art performance only for a subset of these parameters and often on certain anatomic structures. This could hinder the deployment of such models in the clinical setting, as these models might not generalize well when applied to data acquired with different acquisition settings or data acquired from different devices or manufacturers.

The other major limitation of deep learning is interpretability. Traditional machine learning methods offer varying levels of transparency due to the nature of the inputs: features must be carefully selected during training, and the resulting model prediction can be queried against those features. Comparatively, deep learning models are often considered as black boxes. Although there exist methods for visualization of the intermediate representation of neural networks, explainability can also represent an obstacle for unleashing the full potential and widespread adoption of deep learning algorithms in the medical domain.

SUMMARY

In this review, the authors cover the main practical concepts required for understanding and developing deep learning solutions in medical imaging and review the principal deep learning architectures, and general examples of different common categories of applications were provided. They also described the main considerations for training deep learning models. More specifically, underfitting and overfitting and the remedies for addressing these issues are explained. Data imbalance—which is a ubiquitous phenomenon in the medical domain—and how it may affect the performance of deep learning models are also discussed, and some of the solutions for alleviating the effect of data imbalance on the generalizability of deep learning models are specified. Finally, some of the limitations and challenges facing the deployment of deep learning solutions in the clinical setting are mentioned.

Deep learning has opened new horizons in medical image analysis and health care predictive modeling more broadly, and its true potential is still largely untapped. However, for successful development of algorithms that are generalizable and have the potential to be deployed in the health care setting, it is essential to understand the fundamentals as well as pitfalls of this powerful technology.

REFERENCES

1. Silver D, Schrittwieser J, Simonyan K, et al. Mastering the game of Go without human knowledge. Nature 2017;550(7676):354–9.
2. Vinyals O, Babuschkin I, Czarnecki WM, et al. Grandmaster level in StarCraft Ii using multi-agent reinforcement learning. Nature 2019;575(7782): 350–4.
3. Fridman L, Brown DE, Glazer M, et al. MIT autonomous vehicle technology study: Large-scale deep learning based analysis of driver behavior and interaction with automation. arXiv preprint arXiv: 1711.06976 1 (2017).
4. Lin ED, Hefner JL, Zeng X, et al. A deep learning model for pediatric patient risk stratification. Am J Manag Care 2019;25(10):e310–5.
5. McKinney SM, Sieniek M, Godbole V, et al. International evaluation of an AI system for breast cancer screening. Nature 2020;577(7788):89–94.
6. Vaswani A, Shazeer N, Parmar N, et al. Attention is all you need. Adv Neural Inf Process Syst 2017; 5998–6008.

7. Devlin J, Chang M.-W, Lee K, et al. BERT: pre-training of deep bidirectional transformers for language understanding, arXiv preprint arXiv: 1810.04805.

8. Goodfellow I, Bengio Y, Courville A. Deep learning. Cambridge: MIT Press; 2016.

9. Abadi M, Barham P, Chen, J, et al. Tensorflow: A system for large-scale machine learning. In 12th {USENIX} symposium on operating systems design and implementation ({OSDI} 16). Savanah (GA); 2016. p. 265–83.

10. Chollet F. Keras. 2015. Available at: https://github.com/fchollet/keras. Accessed July 29, 2020.

11. Paske A, Gross S, Massa F, et al. PyTorch: An imperative style, high-performance deep learning library. Adv Neural Inf Process Syst 2019;32:8024–35.

12. Chen T, Li M, Li Y, et al. MXNet: A flexible and efficient machine learning library for heterogeneous distributed systems, arXiv preprint arXiv: 1512.01274.

13. JiaY, Shelhamer E, Donahue J, et al. Caffe: Convolutional architecture for fast feature embedding, arXiv preprint arXiv:1408.5093.

14. Manyika J, Chui M, Brown B, et al. Big data: the next frontier for innovation, competition, and productivity, Tech. rep. New York: McKinsey Global Institute; 2011.

15. McCulloch WS, Pitts W. A logical calculus of the ideas immanent in nervous activity. Bull Math Biophys 1943;5(4):115–33.

16. Rosenblatt F. The perceptron: A probabilistic model for information storage and organization in the brain. Psychol Rev 1958;65(6):386–408.

17. Rumelhart DE, Hinton GE, Williams RJ. Learning representations by back-propagating errors. Nature 1986;323(6088):533–6.

18. Deng J, Dong W, Socher R, et al. Imagenet: A large-scale hierarchical image database. IEEE Conference on computer vision and Pattern Recognition, IEEE. Miami (FL), June 20, 2009.

19. Krizhevsky A, Sutskever I, Hinton GE. Imagenet classification with deep convolutional neural networks. In: Pereira F, Burges CJC, Bottou L, et al, editors. Advances in neural information processing systems. Denver (CO): Curran Associates, Inc; 2012. p. 1097–105.

20. Glorot X, Bordes A, Bengio Y. Deep sparse rectifier neural networks. Proceedings of the Fourteenth International Conference on Artificial Intelligence and Statistics. Fort Lauderdale (FL); 2011. p. 315–23.

21. Maas AL, Hannun AY, Ng AY. Rectifier nonlinearities improve neural network acoustic models. Proceedings of the 30th Annual International Conference on Machine Learning, Vol. 30. Atlanta (GA); 2013. p. 3.

22. Rifai S, Vincent P, Muller X, et al. Contractive autoencoders: explicit invariance during feature extraction. Proceedings of the 28th International Conference on International Conference on Machine Learning. Bellevue (WA): ACM; 2011. p. 833–840.

23. Rifai S, Mesnil G, Vincent P, et al. Higher order contractive auto-encoder. Joint European Conference on Machine Learning and Knowledge Discovery in Databases. Athens (Greece): Springer; 2011. p. 645–60.

24. Vincent P, Larochelle H, Bengio Y, et al. Extracting and composing robust features with denoising autoencoders. Proceedings of the 25th International Conference on Machine Learning. Helsinki (Finland): ACM; 2008. p. 1096–1103.

25. Kingma DP, Welling M. Auto-encoding variational bayes, arXiv preprint arXiv:1312.6114.

26. Vincent P, Larochelle H, Lajoie I, et al. Stacked denoising autoencoders: Learning useful representations in a deep network with a local denoising criterion. J Mach Learn Res 2010;11:3371–408.

27. Goodfellow I, Pouget-Abadie J, Mirza M, et al. Generative adversarial nets. Adv Neural Inf Process Syst 2014;27:2672–80.

28. Fan J, Cao X, Xue Z, et al. Adversarial similarity network for evaluating image alignment in deep learning based registration. In: Frangi A, Schnabel J, Davatzikos C, et al, editors. Medical image computing and computer Assisted Intervention – MICCAI 2018. Cham (Switzerland): Springer International Publishing; 2018. p. 739–46.

29. Mahapatra D, Antony B, Sedai S, et al. Deformable medical image registration using generative adversarial networks. 2018 IEEE 15th International Symposium on Biomedical Imaging (ISBI 2018). Washington, DC: IEEE; 2018. p. 1449–1453.

30. Kazeminia S, Baur C, Kuijper A, et al. GANs for medical image analysis, arXiv preprint arXiv:1809.06222.

31. Bi L, Kim J, Kumar A, et al. Synthesis of positron emission tomography (PET) images via multichannel generative adversarial networks (GANs). In: Frangi A, Schnabel J, Davatzikos C, et al, editors. Molecular imaging, reconstruction and analysis of Moving body organs, and stroke imaging and treatment. Cham (Switzerland): Springer International Publishing; 2017. p. 43–51.

32. Yi X, Walia E, Babyn P. Generative adversarial network in medical imaging: A review. Med Image Anal 2019. https://doi.org/10.1016/j.media.2019.101552.

33. Nie D, Trullo R, Lian J, et al. Medical image synthesis with deep convolutional adversarial networks. IEEE Trans Biomed Eng 2018;65(12):2720–30.

34. Frid-Adar M, Diamant I, Klang E, et al. GAN-based synthetic medical image augmentation for increased CNN performance in liver lesion classification. Neurocomputing 2018;321:321–31.

35. Nie D, Trullo R, Lian J, et al. Medical image synthesis with context-aware generative adversarial

networks. In: Frangi A, Schnabel J, Davatzikos C, et al, editors. Medical image computing and computer Assisted Intervention - MICCAI 2017. Cham (Switzerland): Springer International Publishing; 2017. p. 417–25.

36. Cerrolaza JJ, Li Y, Biffi C, et al. 3D fetal skull reconstruction from 2DUS via deep conditional generative networks. In: Frangi A, Schnabel J, Davatzikos C, et al, editors. Medical image computing and computer Assisted Intervention – MICCAI 2018. Springer International Publishing; 2018. p. 383–91.

37. Biffi C, Cerrolaza JJ, Tarroni G, et al. 3d high-resolution cardiac segmentation reconstruction from 2d views using conditional variational autoencoders, arXiv preprint arXiv:1902.11000.

38. Schmidhuber J, Hochreiter S. Long short-term memory. Neural Comput 1997;9(8):1735–80.

39. Cho K, Van Merriënboer B, Bahdanau D, et al. On the properties of neural machine translation: Encoder-decoder approaches, arXiv preprint arXiv:1409.1259.

40. Chung J, Gulcehre C, Cho K, et al. Empirical evaluation of gated recurrent neural networks on sequence modeling. NIPS 2014 Workshop on Deep Learning. Montreal (QC), December 8, 2014.

41. Weiss G, Goldberg Y, Yahav E. On the practical computational power of finite precision rnns for language recognition. Proceedings of the 56th Annual Meeting of the Association for Computational Linguistics (Volume 2: Short Papers). Melbourne (Australia): Association for Computational Linguistics; 2018. p. 740–5.

42. Glorot X, Bengio Y. Understanding the difficulty of training deep feedforward neural networks. Proceedings of the Thirteenth International Conference on Artificial Intelligence and Statistics. Sardinia (Italy): PMLR; 2010. p. 249–56.

43. He K, Zhang X, Ren S, et al. Delving deep into rectifiers: Surpassing human-level performance on imagenet classification. Proceedings of the IEEE International Conference on Computer Vision. Las Condes (Chile): IEEE; 2015. p. 1026–34.

44. Srivastava N, Hinton G, Krizhevsky A, et al. Dropout: a simple way to prevent neural networks from overfitting. J Mach Learn Res 2014;15(1):1929–58.

45. Shorten C, Khoshgoftaar TM. A survey on image data augmentation for deep learning. J Big Data 2019;6(1):60.

46. Nalepa J, Marcinkiewicz M, Kawulok M. Data augmentation for braintumor segmentation: A review. Front Comput Neurosci 2019;13:83.

47. Branco P, Torgo Li, Ribeiro R. A survey of predictive modeling on imbalanced domains. ACM Comput Surv 2016;49(2):1–31.

48. Yang Q, Zhang Y, Dai W, et al. Transfer learning. Cambridge: Cambridge University Press; 2020.

49. Peng J, Kang S, Ning Z, et al. Residual convolutional neural network for predicting response of transarterial chemoembolization in hepatocellular carcinoma from CT imaging. Eur Radiol 2019; 30(1):413–24.

50. Tousignant A, Lemaître P, Precup D, et al. Prediction of disease progression in multiple sclerosis patients using deep learning analysis of MRI data. Proceedings of The 2nd International Conference on Medical Imaging with Deep Learning, Vol. 102. London (UK): MIDL; 2019. p. 483–92.

51. Zhou L, Zhang Z, Chen Y-C, et al. A deep learning-based radiomics model for differentiating benign and malignant renal tumors. Translational Oncol 2019;12(2):292–300.

52. He K, Zhang X, Ren S, et al. Deep residual learning for image recognition. Proceedings of the IEEE Conference on Computer Vision and Pattern Recognition. Las Vegas (NV): IEEE; 2016. p. 770–8.

53. Szegedy C, Vanhoucke V, Ioffe S, et al. Rethinking the inception architecture for computer vision. Proceedings of the IEEE Conference on Computer Vision and Pattern Recognition. Las Vegas (NV): IEEE; 2016. p. 2818–26.

54. Lin T.-Y, Goyal P, Girshick R, et al. Focal loss for dense object detection. Proceedings of the IEEE International Conference on Computer Vision. Venice (Italy): IEEE; 2017. p. 2980–8.

55. Sandler M, Howard A, Zhu M, et al. Mobilenetv2: Inverted residuals and linear bottlenecks. Proceedings of the IEEE Conference on Computer Vision and Pattern Recognition. Salt Lake City (UT): IEEE; 2018. p. 4510–20.

56. He K, Zhang X, Ren S, et al. Identity mappings in deep residual networks. European Conference on Computer Vision. Amsterdam (The Netherlands): Springer; 2016. p. 630–45.

57. Ronneberger O, Fischer P, Brox T. U-Net: Convolutional networks for biomedical image segmentation. International Conference on Medical image computing and computer-assisted intervention. Munich (Germany): Springer; 2015. p. 234–41.

58. Hashemi SR, Prabhu SP, Warfield SK, et al. Exclusive independent probability estimation using deep 3d fully convolutional densenets for isointense infant brain MRI segmentation, arXiv preprint arXiv:1809.08168.

59. Sun J, Yan S, Song C, et al. Dual-functional neural network for bilateral hippocampi segmentation and diagnosis of alzheimer's disease. Int J Comput Assist Radiol Surg 2020;15(3):445–55.

60. Milletari F, Navab N, Ahmadi S.-A. V-net: Fully convolutional neural networks for volumetric medical image segmentation. 2016 Fourth International Conference on 3D Vision (3DV), IEEE, Stanford University, California, October 25, 2016. p. 565–71.

61. Yin S, Peng Q, Li H, et al. Automatic kidney segmentation in ultrasound images using subsequent boundary distance regression and pixelwise classification networks. Med Image Anal 2020;60: 101602.

62. Simonyan K, Zisserman A. Very deep convolutional networks for largescale image recognition, arXiv preprint arXiv: 1409.1556.

63. Chen L, Papandreou G, Kokkinos I, et al. Deeplab: Semantic image segmentation with deep convolutional nets, atrous convolution, and fully connected crfs, arXiv preprint. arXiv:1606.00915.

64. Chen L, Papandreou G, Kokkinos I, et al. Deeplab: Semantic image segmentation with deep convolutional nets, atrous convolution, and fully connected crfs, arXiv preprint arXiv:1606.00915.

65. de Vos BD, Berendsen FF, Viergever MA, et al. A deep learning framework for unsupervised affine and deformable image registration. Med Image Anal 2019;52:128–43.

66. Balakrishnan G, Zhao A, Sabuncu MR, et al. Voxelmorph: A learning framework for deformable medical image registration, arXiv preprint arXiv: 1809.05231.

67. Shen Z, Han X, Xu Z, et al. Networks for joint affine and nonparametric image registration, arXiv preprint arXiv:1903.08811.

68. Eppenhof KAJ, Lafarge MW, Pluim JPW. Progressively growing convolutional networks for end-to-end deformable image registration. In: Angelini ED, Landman BA, editors. Medical imaging 2019: image processing, ociety of Photo-Optical Instrumentation Engineers (SPIE). Bellingham (WA): SPIE Press; 2019. p. 338–44.

69. Yang H, Sun J, Carass A, et al. Unpaired brain MR-to-CT synthesis using a structure-constrained Cycle-GAN, arXiv preprint arXiv:1809.04536.

70. Zhu J.-Y, Park T, Isola P, et al. Unpaired image-to-image translation using cycle-consistent adversarial networks. Proceedings of the IEEE International Conference on Computer Vision. Venice (Italy): IEEE; 2017. p. 2223–2232.

71. Rubin J, Abulnaga SM. CT-To-MR conditional generative adversarial networks for ischemic stroke lesion segmentation. IEEE Int Conf Healthc Inform 2019;(2019):1–7.

72. Bass C, Dai T, Billot B, et al. Image synthesis with a convolutional capsule generative adversarial network. Proceedings of The 2nd International Conference on Medical Imaging with Deep Learning, Vol. 102 of Proceedings of Machine Learning Research. London (UK): PMLR; 2019. p. 39–62.

73. LaLonde R, Bagci U, Capsules for object segmentation, arXiv preprint arXiv:1804.04241.

74. Sabour S, Frosst N, Hinton GE, Dynamic routing between capsules, arXiv preprint arXiv:1710.09829.

75. Sriram A, Zbontar J, Murrell T, et al, GrappaNet: Combining parallel imaging with deep learning for multi-coil MRI reconstruction, arXiv preprint arXiv: 1910.12325.

76. Akagi M, Nakamura Y, Higaki T, et al. Deep learning reconstruction improves image quality of abdominal ultra-high-resolution CT. Eur Radiol 2019;29(11): 6163–71.

77. Gondara L. Medical image denoising using convolutional denoising autoencoders. 2016 IEEE 16th International Conference on Data Mining Workshops (ICDMW). Barcelona (Spain): IEEE; 2016. p. 241–6.

78. Jifara W, Jiang F, Rho S, et al. Medical image denoising using convolutional neural network: a residual learning approach. J Supercomput 2019; 75(2):704–18.

Machine Learning Algorithm Validation

From Essentials to Advanced Applications and Implications for Regulatory Certification and Deployment

Farhad Maleki, PhD[a,1], Nikesh Muthukrishnan, MEng[a,1], Katie Ovens, PhD[b], Caroline Reinhold, MD, MSc[a,c], Reza Forghani, MD, PhD[a,c,d,e,f,*]

KEYWORDS

- Reproducibility • Ability to generalize • Machine learning • Evaluation • Validation
- Cross-validation • Deep learning • Artificial intelligence

KEY POINTS

- Understanding and following the best practices for evaluating machine learning (ML) models is essential for developing reproducible and generalizable ML applications.
- The reliability and robustness of a ML application will depend on multiple factors, including dataset size and variety as well as a well-conceived design for ML algorithm development and evaluation.
- A rigorously designed ML model development and evaluation process using large and representative training, validation, and test datasets will increase the likelihood of developing a reliable and generalizable ML application and will also facilitate future regulatory certification.
- Scalable, auditable, and transparent platforms for building and sharing multi-institutional datasets will be a crucial step in developing generalizable solutions in the health care domain.

INTRODUCTION

With growing interest in machine learning (ML), it is essential to understand the methodologies used for evaluating ML models to achieve reproducible solutions that can be successfully deployed in real-world settings.[1,2] Ability to generalize, meaning that conclusions and algorithms generated based on the specific population studied can be extended to the population at large, is essential for successful translation, deployment, and adoption of ML in the clinical setting. ML is the scientific discipline dealing with developing computational models that can

Funding: R. Forghani is a clinical research scholar (chercheur-boursier clinicien) supported by the Fonds de recherche en santé du Québec (FRQS) and has an operating grant jointly funded by the FRQS and the Fondation de l'Association des radiologistes du Québec (FARQ).

[a] Augmented Intelligence & Precision Health Laboratory (AIPHL), Department of Radiology & Research Institute of the McGill University Health Centre, 5252 Boulevard de Maisonneuve Ouest, Montreal, Quebec H4A 3S5, Canada; [b] Department of Computer Science, University of Saskatchewan, 176 Thorvaldson Bldg, 110 Science Place, Saskatoon S7N 5C9, Canada; [c] Department of Radiology, McGill University, 1650 Cedar Avenue, Montreal, Quebec H3G 1A4, Canada; [d] Segal Cancer Centre, Lady Davis Institute for Medical Research, Jewish General Hospital, 3755 Cote Ste-Catherine Road, Montreal, Quebec H3T 1E2, Canada; [e] Gerald Bronfman Department of Oncology, McGill University, Suite 720, 5100 Maisonneuve Boulevard West, Montreal, Quebec H4A3T2, Canada; [f] Department of Otolaryngology - Head and Neck Surgery, Royal Victoria Hospital, McGill University Health Centre, 1001 boul. Decarie Boulevard, Montreal, Quebec H3A 3J1, Canada

[1] F. Maleki and N. Muthukrishnan contributed equally to this article.

* Corresponding author. Room C02.5821, 1001 Decarie Boulevard, Montreal, Quebec H4A 3J1, Canada.

E-mail address: reza.forghani@mcgill.ca

improve their performance with new experiences. A performance measure, which is defined quantitatively, drives the model building and evaluation process.[3]

Developing a ML model requires 3 major components: representation, evaluation, and optimization.[4] The representation component involves deciding on a type of model or algorithm that is used to represent the association between the input data and the outcomes of interest. Examples of such models are support vector machines, random forests, and neural networks.[5] The evaluation component concerns defining and calculating quantitative performance measures that show the goodness of a representation; that is, the capability of a given model to represent the association between inputs and outputs. Among performance measures that are commonly used for model evaluations are accuracy, precision, recall, mean squared error, and the Jaccard index.[6,7] The aim of the optimization component is to update parameters of a given representation (ie, model) with the goal of increasing the performance measures of interest. Examples of approaches used for optimization are gradient descent–based methods and the Newton method.[8]

In developing ML models, the available data are often partitioned into 3 disjoint sets commonly referred to as training, validation, and test sets. The data from the training set are used to train the model. A model is often trained through an iterative process. In each iteration, a performance measure reflecting the error made by the model when applied to the data in the training set is calculated. This measure is used to update the model parameters in order to reduce the model error when applied to the data in the training set. The model parameters are a set of variables associated with the model, and their values are learned during the training process. Beside model parameters, there might be other variables associated with a model where their values are not updated during training. These variables are referred to as hyperparameters. The optimal or near-optimal values for hyperparameters are determined using data in the validation set. This process is often referred to as hyperparameter tuning. After training and fine-tuning the model, data from the test set are used to evaluate the model for ability to generalize (ie, the performance on unseen data).

This review article first describes the fundamental concepts required for understanding the model evaluation processes. Then it explains the main challenges that might affect the ability to generalize of ML models. Next, it highlights common workflows for evaluation of ML models. In addition, it discusses the implications and importance of a robust experimental design to facilitate future certification and strategies required for deployment of ML models in clinical settings.

ESTIMATING ERROR IN MODEL EVALUATION

In ML applications, available data are often partitioned into training, validation, and test sets. A performance measure is used to reflect the model error when applied to data in these sets. The error made by a model when applied to the data in the training set is referred to as training error, and the error made by a model when applied to data in a test set is referred to as test error. The test error is used as an estimate for the generalization error (ie, the error of the model when applied to unseen data). Therefore, it is essential that data in the test set are not used during training and fine-tuning of the model. Irreducible error, also referred to as Bayes error, is another type of error resulting from the inherent noise in the data. Irreducible error is the lowest possible error achievable for a given task using the available data. This error is independent of the model being used and often cannot be mathematically calculated. It is often estimated by the error made by a group of humans with the domain expertise for the task at hand. The resulting estimate is considered as an upper bound for irreducible error. Understanding these error types is important for developing and evaluating ML models.

Underfitting and overfitting are defined based on the error types described earlier. An underfitted model achieves a training error that is much higher than the irreducible error, and an overfitted model achieves a training error that is much lower than the test error. These concepts are associated with the model complexity; that is, the capacity of a model to represent associations between model inputs and outputs. The complexity of different models can be compared by their number of parameters and the way these parameters interact in the model (eg, linear, nonlinear). Models with high complexity often tend to be too sensitive to the dataset used for training. Often the predictions of a model when trained using different datasets, all sampled from the same population, have a high variance, introducing error. Models with high complexity and consequently high error variance tend to overfit. In contrast, low-complexity models may be biased to learning simpler associations between inputs and outputs that might not be sufficient for representing true associations. For example, a linear model cannot represent an exponential association between inputs and outputs. Low-complexity models tend to underfit.

Developing an optimal model requires a trade-off between bias and variance by controlling model complexity. Also, techniques such as bagging and boosting can be used to control the bias and variance of a model.[9]

As mentioned, the performance on the test set provides an estimation of the generalization error, which indicates the performance of the algorithm on external data. The algorithm's error can be decomposed into 3 terms: irreducible error, estimation bias error, and estimation variance error.[5] The irreducible error, as the name suggests, is irreducible and is caused by noise that usually exists in any test set. The estimation bias and variance are errors caused by the model complexity. Low-complexity models have a high bias and low variance and tend to underfit the training data. Underfitted models typically have a low training performance and low validation and testing performances. In contrast, high-complexity models have a low bias but a high variance and tend to overfit to the training data. An overfitted model typically has a low training error and high validation and testing errors. During model development (ie, before deploying a model on unseen data or a test set), the best method to monitor the performance of a model and its complexity is to observe the error on the training and validation sets and comparing them with the estimate of the irreducible error.[10]

Another factor that should be considered is the choice of a performance measure when evaluating a ML model. For example, consider an application of ML in glioblastoma (GBM) for detecting the pixels corresponding with GBM in a medical image. As shown in **Fig. 1**, the pixels representing the GBM are less than 10% of all pixels in the image, thus, in this example, if an evaluation metric such as global pixel accuracy is used, a learning algorithm may tend toward a naive solution by classifying all pixels as non-GBM to achieve a pixel accuracy of more than 90%. Therefore, the initial goal of learning GBM is obscured because all pixels are considered non-GBM. Suppose a more appropriate metric, such as the Dice score or the Jaccard index, is used instead. In this case, the aforementioned naive solution achieves a score of zero, which prevents the model from suggesting such a naive solution and encourages the model to find solutions that are aligned with the task at hand.

EVALUATION OF MACHINE LEARNING MODELS: TERMINOLOGY

This article uses the following terminology. Training data refers to the data used for learning the model parameters during the training

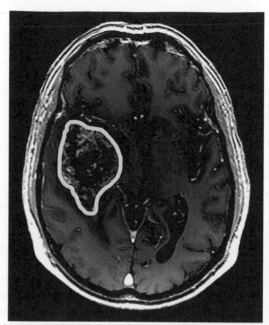

Fig. 1. GBM segmentation example. The pixels in the segmented area inside the yellow contour and corresponding to the heterogenously enhancing mass, are less than 10% of pixels of the image; therefore, care is needed with choosing a relevant performance measure that truly measures performance for GBM pixel recognition rather than an indirect approach (such as global pixel accuracy) tending toward a naive solution based on classifying all pixels as non-GBM.

process. The validation data refers to the data used for searching the optimal set of hyperparameters for a model. The test set refers to the data not being used during the model building (ie, data not being used for model training and fine-tuning).

In ML literature, the terms validation and test have been used interchangeably.[11–13] Furthermore, in medical ML, models can be trained on data from a single or several institutions and evaluated on data from another institution. Although this process is similar to the testing stage in the traditional ML workflow, this form of evaluation has been referred to as external validation,[14–16] and the validation of the model using the local data has been referred to as internal validation.[17,18] This loose terminology causes confusion among researchers. To avoid such confusion, the authors suggest using the terminology in **Table 1**.

MODEL EVALUATION WORKFLOW

Different approaches for ML model validation and evaluation are reviewed here.

Table 1
Suggested terminology for machine learning evaluation

Validation data	Data used for learning hyperparameters or model selection
Test data	Data used for providing an unbiased estimate of the generalization error. Test data should not be used for learning parameters or hyperparameters of the model
Validation error	The error of a model on the validation set. This is not an unbiased estimate of the generalization error. It is used for model selection and fine-tuning of hyperparameters
Test error	An unbiased estimate for the generalization error of a model. Test error is calculated as the model error when applied to test data
Model validation	The process of calculating the validation error for a model
Model evaluation	The process of calculating the test error for a model
Internal evaluation	Model evaluation using the local test data
External evaluation	Model evaluation using the external test data

Holdout Validation

Holdout validation is the most common approach for evaluating ML models (**Fig. 2**). In this approach, the available data is partitioned into training, validation, and test sets.[5] The proportion of the available data used for each set depends on the number of available data points, the data variability, and the characteristics of the model being used. In general, the proportion of the validation

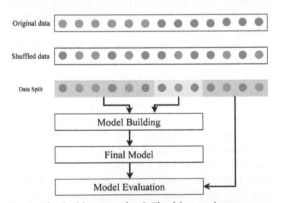

Original data

Shuffled data

Data Split

Model Building

Final Model

Model Evaluation

Fig. 2. The holdout method. The blue and green samples represent different samples from 2 different classes. In the holdout method, samples are randomly assigned to the training (*purple box*), validation (*yellow box*), or test (*orange box*) sets. When the dataset used for training and evaluation of the ML model is small, the performance measures using validation and test sets are sensitive to the composition of these sets, and the resulting performance measures often are not reliable.

set assigned to the training data needs to be large when working with small datasets.[19] Typically, 70% of the available data are used for training, 15% for validation, and the remaining 15% for testing the model, although the percentage allocations can vary.[20] As datasets grow, the ratio between the validation and training sets can be smaller because the validation sets are intrinsically large and better reflect the data.[21] The training and validation sets are used for model building. The data in the training set are used to learn the model parameters. The validation data are used to determine the model hyperparameters during a process called hyperparameter tuning. Although often computationally demanding, hyperparameter tuning can be accomplished in a parallel and automated manner.[22]

Distinguishing between model parameters and model hyperparameters is essential. Model parameters are the model properties (variables) whose values are learned during algorithm training using the training set. For example, weights and bias values in a neural network or the coefficients in a linear regression model are considered parameters. In contrast, hyperparameters are not learned using the training set; the data in the validation set are used to guide the hyperparameter selection. For example, the number of layers in a neural network and the regularization values in a ridge regression model are considered as hyperparameters. Also, the choice of a model, among several different models, is considered a hyperparameter.

After the model is trained and fine-tuned, it is evaluated on the test set to provide an estimate of the model generalization error (ie, the error of the resulting model when applied to unseen data). Therefore, it is essential that the test data are not used during training and fine-tuning the models; otherwise, the estimate for the generalization error would be overoptimistic and unreliable.[23]

The holdout validation approach is commonly used when training deep learning models with large-scale datasets because it is computationally less demanding. However, for small datasets, this approach is criticized for not using the whole dataset. A small test set might not provide a reliable estimate of model performance, and the resulting performance measures might be sensitive to the choice of the test set. For small datasets, selecting a test set large enough to be representative of the underlying data is often impossible. Further, using a larger test set means that fewer samples are available to be used for training the model, which negatively affects the performance of the resulting model. Also, when fine-tuning a model using this approach, the resulting model may be sensitive to the choice of the validation set, resulting in models with low ability to generalize.

Cross-Validation

Cross-validation is a resampling approach used for the evaluation of ML models. The aim of cross-validation is to provide an unbiased estimate of model performance. Compared with holdout validation, this approach tends to provide a more accurate estimate of generalization error when dealing with small datasets. Various cross-validation techniques for the evaluation of ML models are reviewed next.

K-fold cross-validation
In k-fold cross-validation (KFCV), data points are randomly assigned to k disjoint groups (**Fig. 3**). In an iterative process, each time one of these k groups is selected as the validation set, the remaining k − 1 groups are combined and used as the training set. This process is iterated k times so that each group is selected once as the validation set. The average of performance measures across the k iteration is used as the estimate for the validation error. Compared with holdout validation, this approach is computationally more demanding because it requires training and evaluation of the model k times. However, because the model evaluation is performed k times, the variance of the performance measure is reduced and the resulting estimate is more reliable.

The value of k is often chosen such that each of the resulting k groups is a representative sample of the dataset. Another factor that plays a role in determining the value of k is the availability of computational resources. Also, KFCV can be run in parallel to speed up the model evaluation process, which can be accomplished because each iteration of KFCV is independent of the other iterations. The 10-fold and 5-fold cross-validations are the most widely used KFCVs for evaluating ML models.[5]

Stratified k-fold cross-validation
Class imbalance is a common phenomenon in ML. Class imbalance occurs when there is a substantial difference between the number of samples for the majority class and the minority class, where the majority class is defined as the class with the highest number of samples and the minority class is defined as the class with the lowest number of samples. In such a setting, KFCV might lead to unstable performance measures. There might be zero or very few samples from the minority class in 1 or a few of the data folds, which would substantially affect the evaluation metrics for such folds. In the stratified KFCV (SKFCV), each of the k groups of data points are sampled so that the distribution of the classes in each fold closely mirrors the distribution of classes in the whole dataset.

Leave-one-out cross-validation
Although KFCV provides more reliable estimates for generalization error, the resulting model only uses k − 1 groups for training and validation. Leave-one-out cross-validation (LOOCV) uses k = n, where n is the number of samples in the dataset; therefore, all but 1 sample are used for model training. LOOCV is computationally more demanding because it requires training n models. Therefore, it cannot be used when the dataset is very large or the training process for a single model is computationally expensive. LOOCV has been recommended for small or imbalanced datasets.[24]

Leave-p-out cross-validation
Leave-p-out cross-validation (LPOCV) is an extended form of LOOCV, where validation sets can have p elements instead of 1. It is an exhaustive approach designed to use all of the possible validation sets of size p for the evaluation of ML models. For a dataset of n distinct data points, the number of distinct sets of size p, where p = n/k, are as follows:

$$C(n, \ p) = \frac{(n - p + 1) \times \ (n - p + 2) \times \cdots \times n}{1 \times 2 \times \cdots \times (p)}$$

Even for moderately large datasets when p>1, this value exponentially grows, and LPOCV quickly

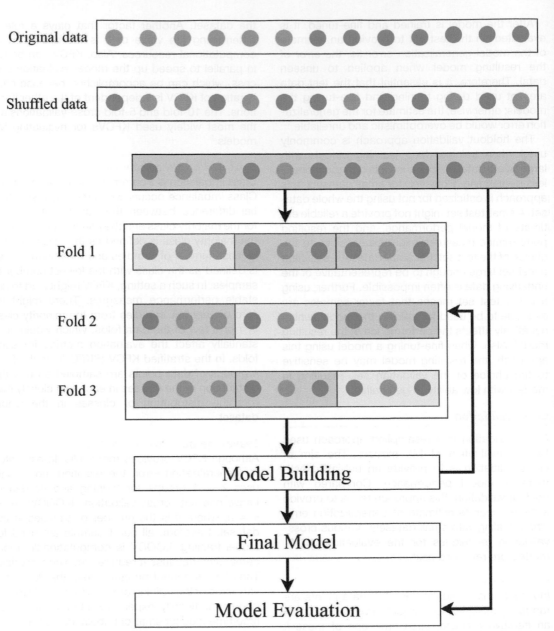

Fig. 3. Three-fold cross-validation (*red bounding box*). In practice, a portion of samples is locked away for calculating an unbiased estimate of the generalization error. The cross-validation method takes the remaining data as input and randomly assigns them to *k* disjoint groups (*k* = 3 in this example). In an iterative process, each time one of these *k* groups is selected as the validation set (*yellow box*) and the remaining *k* − 1 groups are combined and used as the training set (*purple boxes*). This process is iterated *k* times so that each group is selected as a validation set once. The average of the model error on the validation sets then can be used as an estimate of the validation error. Note that, in practice, training and validation data in each iteration are used for learning model parameters as well as selecting hyperparameters for the model. Therefore, the resulting estimate is considered an estimate for the validation error, not for the test error, because the validation data are used for both learning the model parameters and hyperparameters; therefore, it might provide an overoptimistic estimate of generalization error, which is the reason why a test set is locked away before conducting cross-validation. In practice, only in rare cases, such as developing a simple linear regression model that includes a fixed set of variables where the model has no hyperparameters to tune, is a test set not locked away. In such cases, the average of model error (performance measure) on the *k* validation sets can be used as an unbiased estimate of the generalization error (performance measure).

becomes impractical. For small datasets, often a value of p = 2, which is known as leave-pair-out cross-validation, is used to achieve a robust estimate of the model performance.[25] Note that for p = 1, this approach is equivalent to LOOCV.

Leave-one-group-out cross-validation

In some applications, there might be samples in the dataset that are not independent of each other and are somehow related. In such scenarios, the knowledge of one sample from a group might reveal information about the status of other samples in the same group. For example, different pathology slides for the same patients or different MRI scans of a patient during the course of treatment might reveal information about the patient's disease. Having samples from these groups scattered in training, validation, and test sets results in overoptimistic performance evaluations and leads to a lack of ability to generalize. Leave-one-group-out cross-validation (LOGOCV) is similar to LOOCV but, instead of leaving 1 data point out, it leaves 1 group of samples out, which requires that, for each sample in the dataset, a group identifier be provided. These group identifiers can represent domain-specific stratification of the samples. For example, when developing a model for classifying MRI scans into cancerous and noncancerous, all scans for a patient during an unsuccessful course of treatment should have the same group identifier.

Nested cross-validation

Most ML models rely on several hyperparameters. Tuning these hyperparameters is a common practice in building ML solutions. Often, hyperparameter values that lead to the best performance are experimentally sought. In a traditional cross-validation, where data are split into training and validation sets, experimenting with several models and searching for their optimal hyperparameter values often makes the resulting validation error an overoptimistic performance measure if used for estimating generalization error. Therefore, a test set should be locked away and not be used for model training and hyperparameter tuning. The model performance on this test set can be used as a reliable estimate of generalization error. Selecting a single subset of data as the test set for small datasets leads to estimates for generalization error that have high variance and are sensitive to the composition of the test set. Nested cross-validation (NCV) is used to address this challenge (Fig. 4).

NCV consists of an outer cross-validation loop and an inner cross-validation loop. The outer loop uses different train, validation, and test splits.

The inner loop takes a train and validation set chosen by the outer loop, then the model with different hyperparameters is trained using the training set, and the best hyperparameters are chosen based on the performance of the trained models on the validation set. In the outer loop, generalization error is estimated by averaging test error over the test sets in the outer loop. **Fig. 4** shows a 4-fold outer with 3-fold inner NCV.

DATA USED FOR MODEL EVALUATION

Different approaches for model development and evaluation and the impact on algorithm performance were discussed earlier. Here, this article discusses the important attributes of the datasets used for developing reliable ML algorithms.

Data: Size Matters

In some disciplines, developing large datasets for building and evaluating ML models might not be practical. For example, in the medical domain, developing large-scale datasets is often not an option because of the rarity of the phenotype under study, limited financial resources, limited expertise required for data preparation or annotation, patients' privacy concerns, or other ethical or legal concerns and barriers. For example, in the medical imaging domain, experienced physicians are required to manually annotate medical images reliably. Furthermore, because of the patients' privacy concerns and specific legal and regulatory requirements in different jurisdictions, developing a large-scale multi-institutional dataset can be challenging. Therefore, most research is conducted using small datasets. Splitting such small datasets into train, validation, and test sets further shrinks the dataset used for model evaluation, which leads to unreliable estimates of performance measures. Consequently, the resulting models suffer from a lack of ability to generalize and lack of reproducibility.[1] When the dataset used for model building and evaluation is small, the LOOCV or LOGOCV approach is recommended for model evaluation.

If possible, public datasets can be added to the local dataset; however, depending on the structure of a public dataset, there could be an inherent selection bias. Clinicians must be aware of this issue in order to evaluate its impact on the ability to generalize. One example is a mucosal head and neck cancer set consisting mostly of a subset of the disease; for example, human papilloma virus (HPV)–positive oropharyngeal head and neck squamous cell carcinomas (HNSCCs) treated with radiation and chemotherapy. Models trained on such a dataset (eg, for predicting treatment

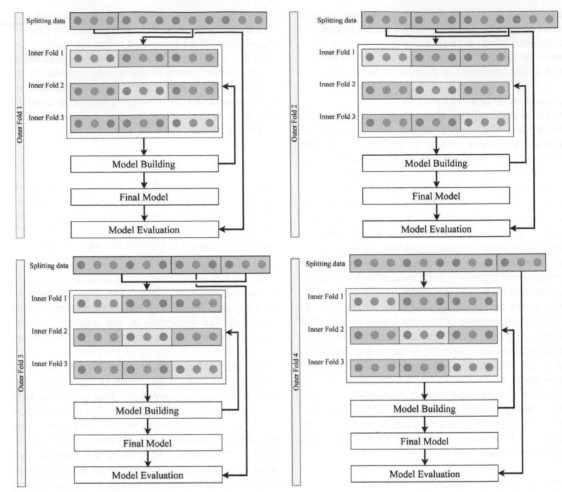

Fig. 4. A 4-fold outer and 3-fold inner NCV. First, the samples in the dataset are randomly shuffled. Then the outer loop uses different train (*purple box*), validation (*yellow box*), and test (*orange box*) splits. The outer folds 1, 2, 3, and 4 are depicted in the top-left, top-right, bottom-left, and bottom-right corners, respectively. For each outer fold, a 3-fold cross-validation highlighted in a red box is used. The model with different hyperparameters is trained using the training set, and the optimal hyperparameters are chosen based on the average performance of the trained models on the validation sets. In the outer loop, generalization error is estimated by averaging test error over the 4 test sets.

response and outcome) may not be generalizable to HNSCCs of the oral cavity, which are typically HPV negative and treated surgically, even though they are still pathologically mucosal HNSCC. The quality of labeling and annotations can also affect model performance. The variability between the public dataset annotations and the annotations in the training data may also lead to models with low ability to generalize.[26] Therefore, data aggregation does not always lead to improving model performance and generalization.[27]

Crowdsourced annotations have also been used to address the challenge of annotating medical datasets.[28–30] Several publications have explored the differences between expert contours and crowdsourced nonexpert contours, which are

generally considered as noisy annotations.[28–30] This research suggests that crowdsourced annotations can translate to improving model performance only with carefully crafted strategies.[28–30]

Another approach commonly used in medical imaging is increasing the number of samples using patch-based approaches.[31] In these approaches, two-dimensional or three-dimensional (3D) patches are extracted from medical images. These patches are then used for model training and evaluation. These approaches often extract several patches from a single image, which leads to increasing the number of available data points for developing and evaluating ML models. For example, instead of treating the GBM example in **Fig. 1** as a single training image, it can be split into several small patches of GBM samples. In such scenarios when the dataset is small, using an LOGOCV approach for model evaluation is recommended to achieve a reliable evaluation of the model performance. Otherwise, the performance measures resulting from this approach might be unreliable and overoptimistic.

Using data augmentation is another alternative for increasing the number of samples used for training and evaluation of ML models. Among examples of commonly used data augmentation techniques are geometric affine transformations such as translation, scaling, and rotation. Data augmentation has been widely used in building ML models for image data, and sophisticated software packages are available for this task.[32,33] However, most of these tools have been designed for regular RGB data (images with three color channels: red, green, and blue) and do not support 3D medical images. Therefore, for 3D images, simple augmentations such as flipping and rotation have been commonly used. Synthetic image generation using generative adversarial networks (GANs) has been also used for data augmentation.[34–38] Although data augmentation is an important tool in developing ML models, proper and impactful application has to be evaluated on a case-by-case basis. When using data augmentation, clinicians must ensure that it is not simply being used to amplify or overrepresent information within the training data, which could result in overfitting.

Data: Variety Matters

Alongside the size of the datasets used for developing and evaluating ML models, the variety in the dataset is a crucial element to consider. Datasets are typically gathered under a variety of circumstances. For example, in medical imaging, scans from different institutions may substantially vary because of factors such as different scanner settings, disease prevalence at a specific institutions because of population demographics, and the use of different protocols. Even within an institution, there are frequently different scanner types, resulting in technical variations, among a list of other potential sources of technical variations and noise. With these factors affecting the data variability, the training, validation, and test sets should represent these variations to be able to create a generalizable model.

Furthermore, because models are selected based on the performance of the validation set, it is crucial that the distribution of the validation set follows the distribution of the test set.[8] If the data distribution of the validation set is different from

that of the test set (eg, validation and test sets are from different institutions or different scanners), the model performance based on the validation set may not translate to a clear picture of model performance for the test set. This situation often manifests as a decline in the model performance measures from the validation set to the test set.

In some medical imaging research, data collected from selected institutions have been used for model building, and the performance of the models has been evaluated using data from a different institution.[14–16] For such models, the performance measures on the test set may not achieve their maximum performance if there is a considerable difference between the distribution of data used for training and data used for evaluating the models.[39] If factors that might substantially affect the data distribution can be controlled, using data from 2 institutions can lead to improving performance measures. In such scenarios, data from the first institution can be used for model development and data from the second institution can be used for model evaluation, which can lead to improving performance measures, because the test set does not need to be held out from the data from the first institution. Therefore, a larger dataset can be used for model building. In addition, this approach does not require sharing the original dataset between institutions, because the trained model in the first institution can be shared with the second institution to be evaluated.

Another important factor that needs to be considered when using data from 1 institution for model development and data from another institution for data evaluation is data representation. Although this approach is considered by many as the gold standard approach for developing a model and evaluating its performance, clinicians need to be aware of the inherent potential pitfalls of this approach. This approach can only be successful if the unique characteristics of evaluation data (eg, from the second institution) are reflected or represented in the training data (eg, from the first institution). If this is not the case, the performance may not be optimal and the generalization error could be overestimated. To make a practical comparison, if an institution is deploying new image analysis software developed based on data from other institutions, the out-of-box algorithm will not perform optimally unless the major characteristics of the scans at the deploying institution are compatible with those used for generating the data used for developing the image analysis software. Using this logic, it also follows that, when deploying an algorithm in a new environment, it may be worthwhile to either evaluate for representation through analyses such as outlier analysis (discussed later) or first perform additional training and validation in the new environment for optimization before deploying the algorithm for use in the new environment.

In addition, certain data samples may be poorly represented in a given dataset. It is important to identify these samples and determine whether they should be excluded or whether more of such samples are necessary in the dataset. Consider a dataset where a small subset of the images are degraded with severe artifacts. Artifacts are common in clinical practice and can be caused by noise, beam hardening from normal anatomic structures, or metal implants. To deploy a generalized model in practice, a model should be able to predict and properly process the image if significant artifact is present; therefore, it is essential that the model is exposed to artifacts in the training and evaluation phases. If images with severe artifact are not well represented, the model may lack the ability to process these cases correctly. To address this issue, a possible approach is the use of preprocessing techniques for artifact reduction as a first step before feeding images to the trained model.[40] In this way, the trained model is treated as a specialized model that is only able to make a prediction or classification in the absence of severe artifact.

To determine whether a sample is poorly represented, techniques that measure the similarity across images in a dataset can be used to identify outliers.[41–43] These techniques use pretrained models to compute feature vectors for each sample in the dataset. Then, similarity scores between all samples are calculated to detect outliers (ie, samples that are different from the rest of the samples in the dataset). Such samples tend to have characteristics that are poorly represented in the dataset. These techniques are also useful to consider when using data from different institutions.[39,44] By identifying outliers or underrepresented samples, samples can be removed from the validation sets to fine-tune performance to a more specific application, or samples similar to the outlier samples can be introduced to the training data to increase confidence in these samples. If a model is designed for working in a specific scenario (eg, only for data with no severe artifact), the limitations of the resulting model must be clearly communicated to avoid using the model in the wrong context. In a deployment setting, such approaches may even be used to flag an image set or scan that may not be well represented and consequently has a high likelihood of not being reliably evaluated by an algorithm. In such cases, the expert radiologist making the final interpretation would be made aware of the potential pitfall, taking this into account for the final interpretation.

IMPLICATION OF ROBUST EXPERIMENTAL DESIGN FOR REGULATORY APPROVAL AND CERTIFICATION

Although a comprehensive discussion of regulatory approval and certification is beyond the scope of this article, optimal algorithm development and evaluation is paramount to successful certification and deployment for patient care in the clinical setting. This article therefore concludes with a brief discussion of this topic. Learning from other industries, such as the pharmaceutical industry, by establishing well-conceived guidelines and ensuring rigorous experimental design from the outset, there is an opportunity to accelerate the future translation of ML algorithms for clinical deployment and use for patient care. The adoption of robust industry-grade platforms that are auditable is also likely to facilitate future certification and clinical deployment.

As interest in ML continues to grow, the widespread deployment of ML models in clinical settings is highly anticipated. The performance of ML models in medical imaging has been shown to achieve performance superior to or comparable with human experts in very selective and controlled settings.[45] In the future, ML models are expected to provide predictions for clinical outcomes of interest and assist clinicians in providing a diagnosis and treatment plan in a timely and accurate manner, enabling more precise and personalized patient therapy and management.[46]

Before deploying a model in a clinical setting, its performance needs to be thoroughly validated and the generalization error needs to be understood. Moreover, if a model is expected to be generalizable, it must have exposure to a variety of samples. Intuitively, data from different institutions may be considered as different distributions based on many factors, including different scanner settings, disease prevalence at a specific institutions caused by population demographics, and following different protocols. This outcome is achieved by carefully considering these factors and their implications, as discussed in this article, to incorporate them into the experimental design.

To properly train generalizable models, large-scale multi-institutional datasets would also be beneficial. Having more data for ML models increases the confidence in predictions and allows robust validation and testing, providing better estimations on the generalization error.[45] Acquiring large-scale datasets is susceptible to its own challenges. Current regulations and infrastructure limitations make data sharing between institutions a tedious and time-consuming process. Furthermore, medical image sets can be large in volume, ranging from several hundred megabytes to several gigabytes, which highlights the need for specialized infrastructures for developing large-scale multi-institutional datasets. Secure cloud platforms that facilitate distributed data access would be ideal for collaboration and building such large-scale multi-institutional datasets. The implementation of scalable and streamlined platforms for data preparation and curation will be a key factor in facilitating the development of reliable ML algorithms in the future.

Before deployment of a ML model in a specific institution, the model needs to be validated within that institution to verify that the model can meet the performance requirements using the local data. Models can also be fine-tuned to the local data to achieve better localized performance, as discussed earlier. However, any changes of a deployed algorithm or its performance need to be excessively examined. Alongside such local validation, ML models generally need to be validated over time as well. For examples, as the prevalence of diseases changes, the deployed models might need to adapt as well. Although ML algorithms can learn from exposure or "experience," the implementation of an actively changing or mutating algorithm for patient care in the clinical setting would be a very complex process that would require robust feedback loops and quality monitoring, ensuring reliable performance and stability, and is unlikely to be the model for implementation in the foreseeable future. Instead, the current model is to develop and evaluate an algorithm using large and varied datasets. The algorithm that is deployed will not be actively changing based on its use after deployment. As such, alternative mechanisms, such as quality monitoring and periodic updates by the vendors based on additional training and evaluation, could be a potential model for optimizing performance in the clinical setting.

Because of the reasons mentioned earlier, algorithms are expected to adapt, and will be required to be accessible, transparent, and auditable. Transparent platforms that allow for continuous evaluation on the performance of an ML model are required to approve the implementation of new ML models or software updates in clinical settings.[47] These platforms should be transparent and auditable such that clinicians can investigate any underlying biases in the datasets or models.[47]

Explainability, to the extent feasible, will also facilitate deployment and adoption. Software pilot programs such as the Precertification Program outlined in the US Food and Drug Administration's Digital Health Innovation Action Plan (https://www.fda.gov/medical-devices/digital-health/digital-health-software-precertification-pre-cert-program) are models that will help the future development of a regulatory framework for streamlined and efficient regulatory oversight of applications developed by manufacturers with a demonstrated culture of quality and organizational excellence. This framework could represent a mechanism through which would-be trusted vendors could deploy artificial intelligence (AI)–based software in an efficient and streamlined manner, including deployment of software iterations and changes, under appropriate controls and oversight. In addition, current regulatory frameworks consider AI algorithms as a software as medical device, which are expected to be locked and not evolving.[48] As experience and comfort with ML applications increases, new regulatory frameworks will have to be developed to allow model adaptations that enable optimal performance while ensuring reliability and patient safety.

SUMMARY

With the surge in popularity of ML and deep learning solutions and increasing investments in such approaches, ML solutions that fail to generalize, when applied to external data, may gain public attention that could hinder the slow but steady adaptation of ML in the health care domain. Following the best practices for the development and evaluation of ML models is a necessity for developing generalizable solutions that can be deployed in clinical settings. This requirement is even more important for deep learning models, which have high capacities and can easily overfit to the available data if a proper methodology for model evaluation is not followed.

Evaluating ML models in the health care domain is often a challenging task because of the difficulty of developing large-scale datasets resulting from the lack of required resources or ethical issues. Because of the small datasets used for development and evaluation of ML models, applications that do not follow a rigorous and sound evaluation procedure are prone to overfitting to the available data. Lack of familiarity with the best practices for model evaluation lead to a lack of generalization of published research. Also, the unavailability of code and data makes evaluating and reproducing such models difficult.

A rigorous experimental design and the use of transparent platforms for building and sharing multi-institutional datasets and following best practices for model evaluation will be crucial steps in developing generalizable solutions in the health care domain. Such platforms could also serve as a medium for reproducible research, which would then increase the likelihood of successful deployment of ML models in the health care domain, with the potential to streamline health care processes, increase efficiency and quality, and improve patient care through precision medicine.

REFERENCES

1. Beam AL, Manrai AK, Ghassemi M. Challenges to the reproducibility of machine learning models in health care. JAMA 2020;323(4):305–6.
2. McDermott MB, Wang S, Marinsek N, et al. Reproducibility in machine learning for health. Paper presented at: 2019 Reproducibility in Machine Learning, RML@ ICLR 2019 Workshop. New Orleans, May 6, 2019.
3. Forghani R, Savadjiev P, Chatterjee A, et al. Radiomics and artificial intelligence for biomarker and prediction model development in oncology. Comput Struct Biotechnol J 2019;17:995.
4. Domingos PM. A few useful things to know about machine learning. Commun ACM 2012;55(10): 78–87.
5. Friedman J, Hastie T, Tibshirani R. The elements of statistical learning, vol. 1. New York: Springer Series in Statistics; 2001.
6. Bertels J, Eelbode T, Berman M, et al. Optimizing the Dice score and Jaccard index for medical image segmentation: Theory and practice. Paper presented at: International Conference on Medical Image Computing and Computer-Assisted Intervention. Shenzhen (China), October 13-17, 2019.
7. Tharwat A. Classification assessment methods. New England Journal of Entrepreneurship 2020. https://10.1016/j.aci.2018.08.003.
8. Goodfellow I, Bengio Y, Courville A. Deep learning. Cambridge (MA): MIT Press; 2016.
9. Quinlan JR. Bagging, boosting, and C4. 5. Paper presented at: AAAI/IAAI, Vol. 1. Portland (Oregon), August 4–8, 1996.
10. Obermeyer Z, Emanuel EJ. Predicting the future—big data, machine learning, and clinical medicine. N Engl J Med 2016;375(13):1216.
11. Erickson BJ, Korfiatis P, Akkus Z, et al. Machine learning for medical imaging. Radiographics 2017; 37(2):505–15.
12. Steyerberg EW, Bleeker SE, Moll HA, et al. Internal and external validation of predictive models: a simulation study of bias and precision in small samples. J Clin Epidemiol 2003;56(5):441–7.
13. Steyerberg EW, Harrell FE. Prediction models need appropriate internal, internal–external, and external validation. J Clin Epidemiol 2016;69:245–7.
14. Kann BH, Hicks DF, Payabvash S, et al. Multi-institutional validation of deep learning for pretreatment identification of extranodal extension in head and neck squamous cell carcinoma. J Clin Oncol 2020; 38(12):1304–11.
15. Welch ML, McIntosh C, Traverso A, et al. External validation and transfer learning of convolutional neural networks for computed tomography dental artifact classification. Phys Med Biol 2020;65(3): 035017.
16. Datema FR, Ferrier MB, Vergouwe Y, et al. Update and external validation of a head and neck cancer prognostic model. Head Neck 2013;35(9):1232–7.
17. König IR, Malley J, Weimar C, et al. Practical experiences on the necessity of external validation. Stat Med 2007;26(30):5499–511.
18. Kocak B, Yardimci AH, Bektas CT, et al. Textural differences between renal cell carcinoma subtypes: machine learning-based quantitative computed tomography texture analysis with independent external validation. Eur J Radiol 2018;107:149–57.
19. Guyon I. A scaling law for the validation-set training-set size ratio. Berkeley (CA): AT&T Bell Laboratories; 1997. p. 1–11.
20. Forghani R, Chatterjee A, Reinhold C, et al. Head and neck squamous cell carcinoma: prediction of cervical lymph node metastasis by dual-energy CT texture analysis with machine learning. Eur Radiol 2019;29(11):6172–81.
21. Guyon I, Makhoul J, Schwartz R, et al. What size test set gives good error rate estimates? IEEE Trans Pattern Anal Mach Intell 1998;20(1):52–64.
22. Hutter F, Kotthoff L, Vanschoren J. Automated machine learning: methods, systems, challenges. Berkeley (CA): Springer Nature; 2019.
23. Russell S, Norvig P. Artificial intelligence: a modern approach. 3rd edition. Upper Saddle River (NJ): Pearson; 2009.
24. Wong T-T. Performance evaluation of classification algorithms by k-fold and leave-one-out cross validation. Pattern Recognition 2015;48(9):2839–46.
25. Airola A, Pahikkala T, Waegeman W, et al. An experimental comparison of cross-validation techniques for estimating the area under the ROC curve. Comput Stat Data Anal 2011;55(4):1828–44.
26. Cohen JP, Hashir M, Brooks R, et al. On the limits of cross-domain generalization in automated X-ray prediction. arXiv preprint arXiv:200202497. 2020.
27. Saha A, Harowicz MR, Mazurowski MA. Breast cancer MRI radiomics: an overview of algorithmic features and impact of inter-reader variability in annotating tumors. Med Phys 2018;45(7):3076–85.

28. Albarqouni S, Baur C, Achilles F, et al. Aggnet: deep learning from crowds for mitosis detection in breast cancer histology images. IEEE Trans Med Imaging 2016;35(5):1313–21.

29. McKenna MT, Wang S, Nguyen TB, et al. Strategies for improved interpretation of computer-aided detections for CT colonography utilizing distributed human intelligence. Med Image Anal 2012;16(6): 1280–92.

30. Nguyen TB, Wang S, Anugu V, et al. Distributed human intelligence for colonic polyp classification in computer-aided detection for CT colonography. Radiology 2012;262(3):824–33.

31. Greenspan H, Van Ginneken B, Summers RM. Guest editorial deep learning in medical imaging: overview and future promise of an exciting new technique. IEEE Trans Med Imaging 2016;35(5):1153–9.

32. Buslaev A, Iglovikov VI, Khvedchenya E, et al. Albumentations: fast and flexible image augmentations. Information 2020;11(2):125.

33. Cubuk ED, Zoph B, Mane D, et al. Autoaugment: Learning augmentation policies from data. arXiv preprint arXiv:180509501. 2018.

34. Zhao H, Li H, Maurer-Stroh S, et al. Synthesizing retinal and neuronal images with generative adversarial nets. Med Image Anal 2018;49:14–26.

35. Salehinejad H, Colak E, Dowdell T, et al. Synthesizing chest x-ray pathology for training deep convolutional neural networks. IEEE Trans Med Imaging 2018;38(5):1197–206.

36. Han C, Kitamura Y, Kudo A, et al. Synthesizing diverse lung nodules wherever massively: 3D multi-conditional GAN-based CT image augmentation for object detection. Paper presented at: 2019 International Conference on 3D Vision (3DV). Québec (Canada), September 16-19, 2019.

37. Frid-Adar M, Diamant I, Klang E, et al. GAN-based synthetic medical image augmentation for increased CNN performance in liver lesion classification. Neurocomputing 2018;321:321–31.

38. Beers A, Brown J, Chang K, et al. High-resolution medical image synthesis using progressively grown generative adversarial networks. arXiv preprint arXiv:180503144. 2018.

39. Storkey A. When training and test sets are different: characterizing learning transfer. Dataset shift in machine learning; 2009. p. 3-28.

40. Philipsen RHHM, Maduskar P, Hogeweg L, et al. Localized energy-based normalization of medical images: application to chest radiography. IEEE Trans Med Imaging 2015;34(9):1965–75.

41. Zhang M, Leung KH, Ma Z, et al. A generalized approach to determine confident samples for deep neural networks on unseen data. In: Greenspan H, Tanno R, Erdt M, et al, editors. Uncertainty for safe utilization of machine learning in medical imaging and clinical image-based procedures. Springer; 2019. p. 65–74.

42. Salimans T, Goodfellow I, Zaremba W, et al. Improved techniques for training gans. Paper presented at: Advances in neural information processing systems. Barcelona (Spain), December 5-10, 2016.

43. Heusel M, Ramsauer H, Unterthiner T, et al. Gans trained by a two time-scale update rule converge to a local nash equilibrium. Paper presented at: Advances in Neural Information Processing Systems. Long Beach (CA), December 4-9, 2017.

44. Glocker B, Robinson R, Castro DC, et al. Machine learning with multi-site imaging data: An empirical study on the impact of scanner effects. arXiv preprint arXiv:191004597. 2019.

45. Miller DD, Brown EW. Artificial intelligence in medical practice: the question to the answer? Am J Med 2018;131(2):129–33.

46. Jiang F, Jiang Y, Zhi H, et al. Artificial intelligence in healthcare: past, present and future. Stroke Vasc Neurol 2017;2(4):230–43.

47. He J, Baxter SL, Xu J, et al. The practical implementation of artificial intelligence technologies in medicine. Nat Med 2019;25(1):30.

48. Shah P, Kendall F, Khozin S, et al. Artificial intelligence and machine learning in clinical development: a translational perspective. NPJ Digit Med 2019;2(1):1–5.

Review of Natural Language Processing in Radiology

Jack W. Luo, MDCM[a], Jaron J.R. Chong, MD, MHI, FRCPC[b],*

KEYWORDS

- Natural language processing • Deep learning • Machine learning • Radiology • Artificial intelligence

KEY POINTS

- Natural language processing (NLP) will enable a variety of assistive radiologic applications.
- Advances building on NLP techniques will permit machines to understand, classify, summarize, and generate text to automate linguistic tasks.
- NLP algorithms can be complementary to other radiology imaging artificial intelligence applications for diagnostic or workflow enhancement.

INTRODUCTION

In computer vision, breakthrough performance in 2012 for image classification using deep learning–based AlexNet has caused a frenzy in neural networks.[1] In recent years, radiology has embraced the potential of deep learning–based computer vision systems to enhance clinical diagnosis and improve the efficiency of the modern radiology workflow, automate detection, and extend the clinical prognostic capabilities of radiologists and physicians alike.

In contrast, natural language processing (NLP) has seen lesser coverage from the radiology artificial intelligence community. However, the application of machine learning, including deep learning techniques in NLP, among many other fields, has led to substantial improvements across a variety of NLP tasks. These tasks include, but are not limited to, text classification, speech recognition, machine translation, and automatic summarization.[2–4] These aforementioned tasks all have downstream applications, whether direct or indirect, to the practice of a clinical radiologist, because report creation is a central component of a radiologist's job. As such, there is a growing need for radiologists to understand not only the latest technologies driving image interpretation but also those driving text understanding and generation.[5]

In this article, key components of modern NLP are covered. Common preprocessing techniques such as tokenization and lemmatization are reviewed. This article covers the use of word embeddings as a tool to abstract meaning and explore the use of classic machine learning techniques and deep learning for NLP tasks. In addition, it discusses clinical applications of NLP and provides future directions for its use in radiology.

WHAT IS NATURAL LANGUAGE PROCESSING?

NLP is defined as a branch of artificial intelligence that is concerned with the interaction between computers and humans using natural language. NLP is a multidisciplinary field that combines classic linguistics with traditional computer science and modern artificial intelligence (AI) methods. The intention of NLP is to enable machines to read and understand human languages for meaningful purposes. Given the diversity of tasks possible, there are potentially many different

a Department of Radiology, McGill University, 1001 Decarie Boulevard, Room B02.9375, Montreal, QC H4A 3J1, Canada; b Department of Medical Imaging, Western University, 800 Commissioners Road East, Room C1-609, London, ON N6A 5W9, Canada
* Corresponding author.
E-mail address: jaron.chong@lhsc.on.ca

Neuroimag Clin N Am 30 (2020) 447–458
https://doi.org/10.1016/j.nic.2020.08.001

customizations or workflows possible, which at first glance can seem significantly more abstract that the concepts and technologies that drive computer vision applications. However, as personal familiarity with various workflows grows, there are certain patterns that emerge common to any natural language application. Similar to image analysis methods, there are, broadly, the stages of (1) preprocessing, which can use both classic or word-embedding methods to convert raw data into a format suitable for machine learning; and (2) model training, which can use either classic machine learning or deep learning methods, toward the broad task categories of language understanding or generation.

Preprocessing

Converting raw text into a format usable for training language models often requires many preprocessing steps. In NLP terminology, individual radiology reports, individual medical charts, or any other raw-text file is commonly referred to as a document, and a collection of documents, such as a collection of radiology reports, is referred to as a corpus. Similar to computer vision and imaging workflows, many NLP workflows rely on a common set of preprocessing tasks to convert raw data into a format suitable for model training and machine learning.

Tokenization and Stop Words

Tokenization is defined as the conversion of words into an indexed format (Fig. 1). Said index can be derived from either a predefined vocabulary (eg, a list of all English words) or, more typically, from all the words in a defined corpus. In common practice, that indexed format is stored in a vector where the unit corresponds to the index position. For instance, if "alphabet" is the first word in the index, and "radiology" is the second, and "steeple"

<No acute cardiopulmonary abnormality.>

↓

```
SentenceTokenizer
```

<no> <acute> <cardiopulmonary> <abnormality> <.>

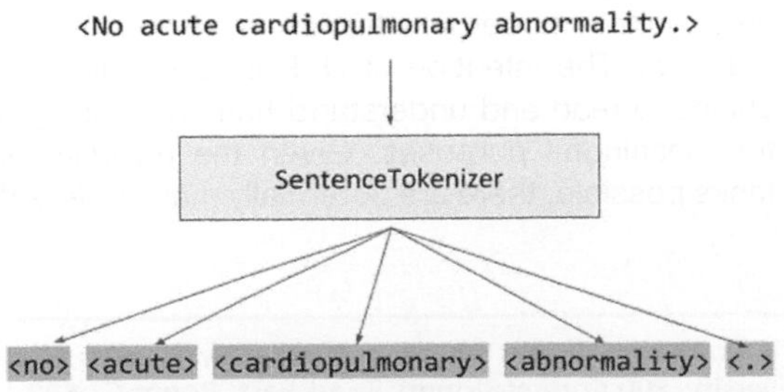

Fig. 1. String array tokenization. Individual words in a string are converted into indexed tokens. The final vectorized string represents the original string numerically, with tokenized numbers representing each word.

the third, radiology would be converted as [0, 1, 0], alphabet as [1, 0, 0], and steeple as [0, 0, 1].[6] Tokenization or vectorization of language accomplishes multiple aims, on a practical level, compressing complex documents into a condensed representation saving computation memory and processing power, but, at a linguistic level, also assists in the conceptual abstraction of vocabulary, combining closely related keywords or disambiguating words that can have multiple meanings.

Commonly, particularly when dealing with unstructured raw full text, certain small words are deliberately omitted and not tokenized. These excluded words, a concept known as stop words, refer to particularly common words that may not contribute significant information to the desired task, such as "the," "a," "is," and "on." By eliminating such words, space is saved and subsequent model training can be accelerated. In many cases, model performance is also increased as stop-word removal permits a model to ignore irrelevant vocabulary.[7]

Note that, for certain tasks, a poor choice of stop words may eliminate valuable contextual information from a document, particularly negations (eg, "no," "not") and a high frequency of a keyword does not necessarily imply a lack of utility. Furthermore, in the process of tokenization, minor differences in capitalization or other forms of character representation and language may be intentionally ignored, improving model performance. For instance, "EMBOLUS," "embolus," and "Embolus" would be abstracted to the same keyword token.

Stemming and Lemmatization

Given the diversity of keywords, occasionally, an additional preprocessing step is performed, known as lemmatization or stemming. In both approaches, words such as "walking" and "talking" and "radiologically" would be reduced to "walk," "talk," and "radiology." Lemmatization differs from stemming in that it attempts to reduce the words to a proper lemma (ie, a base word that can be found in the dictionary), and thus takes into proper context and semantic meaning, and in the process performs a dimension reduction or abstraction of a word to a high-level concept.[8] Between the 2 concepts, lemmatization is a more rigorous technique and can perform complex, nonintuitive abstractions, such as reducing the word "better" to "good," 2 words that are conceptually related, but spelt differently from one another and have few characters in common. In comparison, stemming purely functions via pattern matching, crudely truncating the ends of words according to a predetermined rule set (eg, removing "-ing" from verbs "talking" to "talk"). Occasionally, this can result in errors known as overstemming or understemming. For example, with overstemming, a stemmer may stem the words "universal," "university," and "universe" to "univers-," inadvertently combining 3 words to 1 stem concept despite how unrelated the 3 original words are. Although stemming can miss edge cases handled by lemmatization, it is much faster than lemmatization and is thus more commonly used.[9]

Parts-of-Speech Tagging

Parts of speech (POS) refers to the grammatical function each word has in a sentence. Nouns, pronouns, adjectives, verbs, prepositions, conjunctions, and interjections are all considered POS classes. The identification of individual POS in a sentence is referred to as POS tagging.[10]

Given that the same word can have different meanings in different contexts, POS tagging can extract additional salient information available not directly from the word itself but from its relation within a sentence. For instance, the word "answer" in "Give me your answer" is a noun, whereas, in the sentence "Answer the question," the word "answer" is a verb. POS tagging can thus be the first step toward word sense disambiguation, which refers to the act of distinguishing between different meanings for the same word given a context.[11]

Bag of Words and N-Grams

The concept of bag of words simply refers to the representation of a text as an unordered set of its component words. Such an approach simplifies storage, because context and grammar are ignored, but word frequency is kept.[12] As such, if a document's text is "the apple is a red apple," a bag-of-words model would represent it as ["apple", "apple", "the", "is", "a"], or, if common stop words are removed, ["apple", "apple"]. However, the lack of word context is problematic, especially when dealing with large documents or sentence structure. A more advanced formulation, bigram and trigram models, attempts to provide close-range context by taking into account 1 or 2 consecutive neighbors respectively before conversion into a bag-of-words representation.[13] Under a bigram model, the preceding document would be stored as [(the, apple), (apple, is), (is, a), (a, red), (red, apple)]. The usage of such N-gram models can help preserve greater amounts of contextual information, although, in

practice, representations more than trigram are seldom used.

Term Frequency–Inverse Document Frequency

Term frequency–inverse document frequency [TF-IDF] is a numerical statistic intended to rank how important or not important a word is in a given document. The dual concepts of term frequency and inverse document frequency contribute to that score. Term frequency, a more intuitive concept, measures the frequency of a word in a given document. Although this offers a certain degree of proportionality, with more frequent keywords having a high relevance score, this can quickly permit very frequent but unimportant words (eg, "the," "and") to seem to be overly relevant. In contrast, inverse document frequency measures the number of documents that contain the term at least once for a given corpus, which allows for the down-weighting of common terms that appear in nearly all documents.[14]

By multiplying term frequency with inverse document frequency, the TF-IDF score is obtained. A term with high TF-IDF would be one that appears frequently in a single document (eg, "subarachnoid" in the case of a brain report) but not frequently across all documents in a corpus (eg, all radiological reports). TF-IDF is an important concept not only with search queries and document search but also with NLP machine learning and AI models because the use of a TF-IDF value can provide relative weighting and importance of a given keyword in a document or corpus.

Negation Detection

Negation detection is the act of identifying cues that imply a negative sentiment (eg, "no evidence of," "no longer seen," "has resolved"), with a particularly important role to play with respect to patient cohorting, particularly for research and quality assurance workflows.[15] Although identification of findings and diseases can be achieved using keyword matching, distinguishing between the presence or absence of disease in a report requires accurate negation detection. Because of the variety of possible ways to phrase a negation sentence, this can be a challenging task unto itself. Very early rules-based attempts to perform this task, most notably a regular expression algorithm called NegEx showed early success at performing this task in biomedical documents,[16] but quickly encountered limitations with respect to false-positives caused by failures to take into account dependency relationships between keyword concepts and negation words. Multiple efforts since then have attempted to improve the accuracy of such systems with more advanced incorporation of POS tags and syntactic analysis through parsing of the grammatical tree.[17]

WORD EMBEDDINGS
Definition

Although simple tokenization of words allows the mapping of each individual word to an index as a one-dimensional array or vector, those tokenization approaches miss the context 2 similar words might have with one another. For instance, a model that assigns a numerical index to a word based on alphabetical position might place "king" and "queen" or "men" and "women" very far apart, but these terms have closely related higher-level concepts (ie, "royal titles", "gender").

Instead of simply translating words into a machine-readable format the way tokenization alone does, word embedding tries to capture the semantic and contextual information inherent in the vocabulary. By encoding words into vectors where the distance and direction measures its semantic relationship instead of being arbitrary, vector operations can be performed on those terms, thus allowing the model to understand the relative meaning of one word versus another.[18]

By doing so, the model gains a proper semantic understanding of the words, and thus obtains a mathematical representation of synonyms, analogies, and modifier words. Typically, the use of word embeddings results in substantial improvements in model performance (**Fig. 2**).

Word2vec and GloVe

One of the most common word embedding models is Word2vec, which was published in 2013 by an NLP team at Google.[18] Word2vec, using a shallow 3-layer neural network, attempts to either predict the context of any given word given the center word (skip-gram) or to predict the center word given a series of context words (continuous bag of words).

For instance, words such as "hemorrhage" can occur either in the context of "subarachnoid hemorrhage," "intraparenchymal hemorrhage," or "intraventricular hemorrhage." Thus, the words "subarachnoid," "intraparenchymal," and "intraventricular" would be classified into the same category, and thus be close to one another in the vector space, because all 3 words frequently occur with the word "hemorrhage." As such, other words close to these 3 will likely refer to other layers of the neuroanatomy as well.

Although Word2vec generates embeddings using a predictive neural network–based model, GloVe, in contrast, directly uses the co-occurrence matrix of all words in a given corpus to generate individual word embeddings following dimensionality reduction techniques.[19] In practice, GloVe embeddings are typically easier to obtain than Word2vec and perform better on semantic relatedness tasks such as analogies, but they usually take much more memory to store. However, neither the Word2vec nor the GloVe approach works well with dealing with out-of-vocabulary words if the embeddings are derived from a small corpus (**Fig. 3**).

For reasons concerning both performance and ability to generalize, off-the-shelf embedding models are typically trained on large corpora of publicly available texts such as Wikipedia. In recent years, there have been attempts to train radiology-specific word embeddings with a corpus derived from free-text reports, such as the Intelligent Word Embeddings initiative, which uses a Word2vec-derived model.[20]

RULES-BASED AND CLASSIC MACHINE LEARNING TECHNIQUES
Regular Expressions

Regular expressions, additionally termed as regex or regexp is a sequence of characters that define a search pattern, often used for searching and matching patterns found in strings. Although more commonly known whole search keyword matching is encompassed within the functionality of regular expressions, the concept and syntax of regular expressions is an extremely compact but expressive manner in which to compose matching rules for strings. Originating from theoretic works on regular languages and mathematics

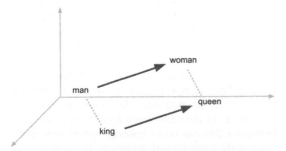

Fig. 2. Word vector embeddings. Models can be generated to map a set of words or phrases to vectors of numerical values, and to reduce the high dimensionality of words into a learned lower dimensional representation. In the process of deriving this embedding, derived vectors can sometimes derive fundamental concepts and linguistic structures; for example, as depicted, the relationship between gender and a title.

X=

	There	is	no	evidence	of	pulmonary	embolus	.
There	0	2	1	0	0	0	0	0
is	2	0	0	1	0	1	0	0
no	1	0	0	2	0	0	1	0
evidence	0	1	2	0	1	0	0	0
of	0	0	0	1	0	0	0	1
pulmonary	0	1	0	0	0	0	2	1
embolus	0	0	1	0	0	2	0	1
.	0	0	0	0	1	1	1	0

Fig. 3. Co-occurrence matrix. A co-occurrence matrix represents the number of times a word appears in the same context as another word. Higher values of co-occurrence may reflect natural relationships and structure between certain words (eg, "no evidence," "pulmonary embolus").

from 1951,[21] regular expressions entered popular use in 1968 with early applications in pattern matching in text editors and lexical analysis in computer source code compilation,[22,23] and have proved to be a foundational concept, continuing to be an essential part of the standard libraries of many modern programming languages.

Many well-defined NLP tasks are surprisingly enabled by the smallest regular expressions, particularly in circumstances in which vocabulary is well defined and the variations in expression are few. One of the most highly cited negation detection algorithms, NegEx, used a regular expression crafted to detect an exhaustive list of negative phases ranging from [no, not, without, ruled out] to more advanced phrases such as [no sign of, not demonstrate, no evidence of] with incorporation of flexible word proximity to account for multiple phrase variations of phrases (eg, "{No} {pulmonary embolus}," "{No}evidence of {pulmonary embolus}").[16]

Naive Bayes, Support Vector Machines, and Random Forests

At first glance, it may seem improbable that classic machine learning techniques, many of which are numeric, would have much linguistic application. However, leveraging tokenization and vectorization preprocessing enables the numerical analysis of documents. Once converted into a numeric vector, in effect, the training of the machine learning model is amenable to statistical and machine learning modeling, with the model learning the associations between an input vector and the desired output. This model of analysis works best when considering tasks involving document classification or sentiment analysis but can be extended to other more advanced tasks, such as POS tagging and named-entity recognition.

Classic NLP machine learning techniques rely on training a supervised learning model to generate classifications given input vectors, which could range from a binary naive Bayes classifier for keywords and POS to more complex models involving large dimension input vectors to support vector machines, or random forests (**Fig. 4**). Through the combination of relative word N-gram frequencies with naive Bayes, random forest decision rules, or support vector machine separation hyperplanes on the input vectorized string, classifications can be made to support the desired NLP task.[24]

Deep Learning

Deep learning refers to a more contemporary subtype of machine learning that is able to better able to exploit greater quantities of raw, structured, and unstructured data to derive higher-level representations of information, accomplishing this by using neural networks with vastly greater layers and parameter spaces than previously thought trainable, and exploiting novel methods of training to permit successful model generation. In practice, almost all deep learning models are now implemented using neural networks, an architecture consisting of interconnected nodes, or neurons, inspired by, but distinct from, human neuronal architecture.[25] A detailed review of deep learning is provided in a separate article in this issue, but a brief overview is provided here.

Convolutional Neural Networks

A particularly successful architecture in computer vision and medical imaging is that of the

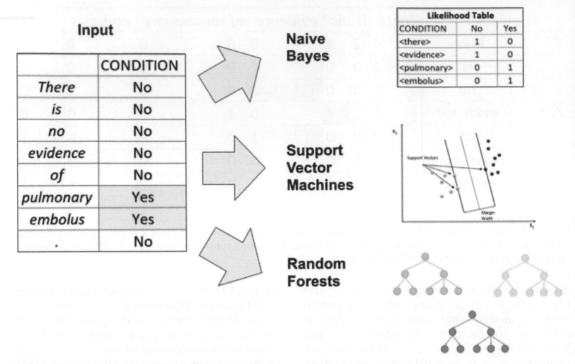

Fig. 4. Classic machine learning; naive Bayes, support vector machines, random forests. String arrays and tokens can be converted into a vectorized representation with desired output classifications. Depending on the specific machine learning method used, a frequency and likelihood table may be calculated with naive Bayes, support vectors, and hyperplanes determined with support vector machines, or decision rules generated for random forests in order to perform the desired classification task.

convolutional neural network (CNN). CNNs, also known as convnets, are a type of neural network that relies on mathematical operations called convolutions. A convolution refers to the application of a filter to a contiguous number of points around a central input point. In the case of imaging, convolutions can be used for sharpening or blurring a two-dimensional input (the image) around a specific (eg, 5×5) window. A CNN (**Fig. 5**) integrates multiple convolutional nodes or neurons into a neural network and is the architecture responsible for breakthrough performance on a variety of image classification and object detection tasks.[26]

Although CNNs have encountered great success within imaging, it may not be immediately intuitive, but text processing can benefit from a convolutional approach as well. In contrast with the bag-of-words approach, which encodes a document as a sum of its words, a CNN approach for text treats the input as a vector and thus applies convolutional operations around a center word. By doing so, the model is able to learn the local context of any given word depending on the filter size: a filter of length 7 would learn a word with 3 neighbor words before and after,

similar to how, in imaging, a 7×7 filter would train on a 7×7 pixel region on an image (**Fig. 6**).

As such, a CNN approach to NLP understands the local context for any word in a given sentence. Through second-order convolutions (eg, paragraph level, sentence level) stacked on first-order (eg, word level) convolutions, and so on, the model can cover larger and larger parts of a document until it is fully covered. The hierarchical representation of words in a CNN allows the model to get a global understanding of any given document.[27]

In practice, combined with the latest word embedding techniques such as Word2vec, CNNs have obtained good performance across a variety of NLP tasks, in particular in the task of document classification.

Recurrent Neural Networks and Long Short-Term Memory

Another popular type of neural network architecture is that of a recurrent neural network (RNN). In traditional network architectures, including CNNs, current inputs are independent of past inputs or outputs. In contrast, RNNs are a particular

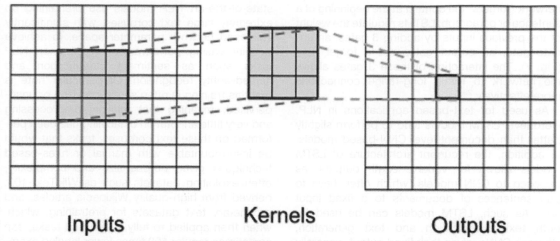

Inputs   Kernels   Outputs

Fig. 5. Deep learning CNNs. Simplification of CNNs. An input array is convolved using a kernel to a higher-level output array. Through multiple layers of convolutions, the input information is increasingly abstracted toward a desired outcome. Although depicted as a two-dimensional array visually, this is arbitrary, and convolutions can occur at 1 dimension or higher arbitrary N dimensions.

form of neural networks in which the output from a previous step is fed as an input to the current step, in addition to the current input. This architecture explicitly allows the modeling of sequencelike structures, such as text or time-series data.[28] As such, although CNNs can only process single data points such as an image or a full document, RNNs can process sequences of data, such as sentences or a stream of data from a biologic hardware sensor. An RNN-based model can more naturally handle individual words in a sentence, as opposed to whole documents. A particularly well-performing RNN architecture, because of its robustness, is a long short-term memory (LSTM) network. Traditional RNNs typically perform poorly with long sequences because of the way neural networks are trained, leading to a problem known as vanishing gradient, where a

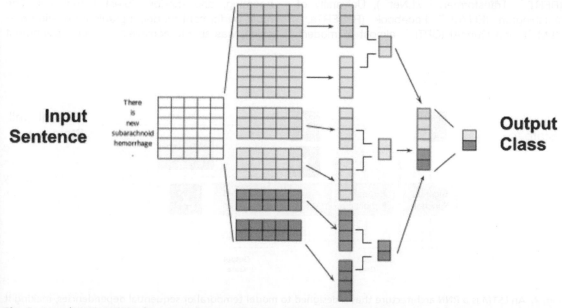

Input Sentence   There is new subarachnoid hemorrhage .   Output Class

Fig. 6. Deep learning CNNs for sentiment classification. CNN modeling of context converting an input sentence, which, through a series of convolutional operations, outputs 2 output classes, for example, in a positive diagnosis sentiment classification task.

network "forgets" the context at the beginning of a sentence or paragraph. LSTMs regulate the weight of the previous inputs by adding 3 gates: an update gate, an output gate, and a forget gate (Fig. 7). The interaction of these 3 gates allows the network to retain long-range connections more effectively.[29]

As used for text-based applications in NLP, word-level LSTM models tend to perform slightly better than document-level CNN-based models. In addition, the recurrent architecture of LSTM models allows for variable-length outputs, as opposed to CNN models, which often have to pad sentences of documents to a fixed input size. As such, LSTM models can be used for both text classification and text generation, whereas CNNs, given their fixed output, generally only perform classification. However, a major downside for recurrent models is that they are more difficult and more computationally resource intensive to train than CNN models and less parallelizable. LSTM models can often be slower by at least 1 to 2 orders of magnitude.[30]

Semisupervised, Transfer Learning, and Transformer Based Natural Language Processing Approaches

Since 2018, there has been substantial innovation with NLP techniques, by exploiting ideas that have proved critical to performance with image-based tasks. Beginning with ULMFiT,[31] with leading efforts from leading AI laboratories such as Google (BERT,[32] Transformer,[33] XLNet[34]), University of Washington (ELMo),[35] Facebook (RoBERTa,[36] XLM[37]), and OpenAI (GPT),[38] almost all modern state-of-the-art NLP models use pretraining on extremely large text corpuses, with significantly increased network parameter space, to achieve ever-increasing performance on common NLP tasks such as sentiment classification and named-entity recognition. Of particular note is that this training is often semisupervised or unsupervised, meaning that minimal preprocessing and very little annotation or labeling has been performed on these text corpuses, tasks that would be insurmountable with manual or rules-based techniques given corpus size and complexity, often exploiting datasets such as WikiText-103, derived from high-quality Wikipedia articles, and proprietary text datasets for pretraining, which, when then applied to fully supervised tasks, can sometimes require 100 times fewer labeled examples to achieve comparable performance. This point is of particular interest to radiology and biomedical applications given the significant variety and difficulty required to complete labeling.

CLINICAL APPLICATIONS
Automatic Protocoling

Some investigators have proposed using machine learning to automate magnetic resonance (MR) imaging protocol selection of radiology requisitions. In a study by Brown and Marotta,[39] a machine learning model was developed to classify unstructured clinical history indications and assign MR imaging protocols, with attempted models comparing support vector machine, gradient boosting, and random forest techniques. The most performant model, a gradient boosting machine, was able to achieve a protocol assignment

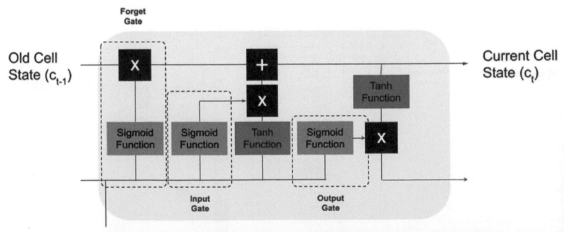

Fig. 7. An LSTM is a RNN architecture that is designed to model temporal or sequential dependencies, making it highly relevant for usage in NLP. Its primary advantage is its ability to inform current state predictions using information from prior states using memory cells, enabling this network design to capture long-range language dependencies.

accuracy of 95%. More advanced NLP methods for performance of the same task have been proposed to permit comprehensive MR imaging and computed tomography (CT) protocoling using more advanced Word2vec models.[40]

Extraction of Language Features, Patient Cohorting, and Coded Ontology from Charts

There has been a significant amount of attention paid within the informatics and electronic health record community to the ability of NLP to perform extraction of details from medical records and narrative text, particularly with regard to tasks of statistical data collection, insurance billing, and patient cohorting.[41,42] NLP has been used to screen large databases of radiographs to identify patients with conditions for study enrollment, which has been shown to rival and sometimes be superior to traditional discharge note coding.[43] In addition, such systems have been shown to perform better in document corpora in which there is standardized formatting and terminology, such as with BI-RADS (Breast Imaging-Reporting and Data System) assessment categories, supporting continuing clinical efforts to increased structured reporting in clinical practice.[44]

Medical Imaging Appropriate Use and Clinical Follow-up, and Diagnostic Yield

Similar technologies to patient abstraction have been proposed to directly monitor and influence referring physician ordering, follow-up recommendations, and appropriate use of medical imaging resources. In an article from Dang and colleagues,[45] an online processing workflow was devised to process recommendations made in greater than 4 million radiology reports over a 10-year period to identify reports with and without follow-up recommendations. The system was able to identify different trends between examinations in which there were greater amounts of recommendations, which could vary by age and imaging modality. In a more recent article by Santo and colleagues[46] (2016) evaluating the effectiveness of a monitoring system to identify lack of follow-up for abdominal imaging findings suspicious for cancer, a more comprehensive system was devised that attempted to short-list and identify clinically significant incidental findings and recommendations, following which an attempt to directly contact referring physicians was made to ensure awareness of findings. In 1 out of 10 patients, the monitoring system was able to identify inappropriate lack of follow-up, providing a valuable process to navigate poor handoffs in care and follow-up

examination scheduling. Similar concepts have been proposed for other diseases and conditions, including sentiment classification of pulmonary embolus, with calls for deploying similar techniques in providing appropriate-use feedback to referring clinicians.[47,48]

Summarization of Patient Dossiers

The effective practice of radiology often requires the integration of clinical contextual information with radiologic imaging findings. With the rapid adoption of the electronic medical record, reviewing and assimilating preceding clinical information, and findings from multiple prior imaging studies can be challenging, the need for which will continue to increase as the length of electronic health records grows. NLP techniques have been proposed that could automatically not only extract diseases and conditions but also generate a summarized report to rapidly familiarize a radiologist with findings from prior clinical records and radiology reports.[49] Such summarization techniques have also been proposed to aid in the abstraction of measurements and descriptors to pretabulate lesion measurements from prior CT and MR imaging reports to aid in tracking lesions over multiple radiologic encounters.[50]

Conversational Interfaces

At the extreme end of NLP are text generative interfaces, capable of conversing and answering questions for specific indications, often even directly with patients. In a recent article by Chetlen and colleagues[51] (2019), chatbot technology was used to educate patients before breast biopsy. Delivered via a touch-screen tablet given to patients just before undergoing a breast biopsy procedure, by sampling a large query of more than 5000 forum thread conversations from breast cancer treatment center Web sites, a statistical model was created to create a condensed list of questions and answers, which was presented to patients in a conversation interface. In patient survey testing toward the chatbot, 18 (33%) women strongly agreed and 29 (54%) agreed that the chatbot made it easier to understand their procedure, with most agreeing that it improved their quality of care.

LIMITATIONS

Working with NLP poses different challenges and obstacles in comparison with machine learning in computer vision, some of which are unique to linguistics. One key difficulty when working with NLP problems concerns the accessibility of training datasets. In contrast with the longer open-science public record of recent machine learning and AI competitions and imaging datasets, because of the inherently private nature of reports and biomedical text, large public datasets of medical records rivalling the size of a Wikipedia corpus or public Internet corpus are not commonly available and, for health care organizations, are extremely difficult to extract and release given the significant difficulty of ensuring text anonymization. The persistence of free narrative reporting and interpractitioner differences also makes model training difficult, particularly with respect to the ability to generalize language models between divisions and hospitals, which may have unique vocabulary, expressions, or terminology. Even if existing language ontologies are leveraged, these may not be localized to a particular environment and often require significant customization to produce performant results rivalling research systems. In addition, there are inherent limitations to NLP-based approaches with respect to patient cohorting and labeling, which are fundamentally limited by the degree of specificity and detail available in routine clinical notes and reports, which are often written for reasons of only facilitating appropriate clinical care, and not to the level of detail required for machine learning applications development.

SUMMARY

The ability to generalize with machine learning and AI technologies permits a wide gamut of possibilities and applications. Although much attention has been paid to image interpretative tasks, numerous other opportunities exist with NLP that offer similar or greater clinical value, often as an adjunctive or assistive technology, which could lead to improved clinical workflows, greater safety and efficiencies, and improved patient quality of life and health care satisfaction. Rather than posing an existential threat to radiologists, many of these applications are inherently complementary, freeing radiologists from mundane or routine tasks. Some investigators have suggested that NLP radiology informatics applications to potentially be "low-hanging fruit" of radiology AI, far more feasible and practical than automation of imaging diagnosis, with workflow transformations realizable immediately. In addition, there are many who see NLP as a necessary complement and enabling precursor to image interpretation AI tasks, particularly with respect to patient cohorting to permit AI model development of every disease and condition. Behind every medical imaging examination is a radiologic report, 2 sides of the

same truth, with NLP perhaps playing an essential role, in unlocking the possibilities of radiology AI.

DISCLOSURE

J.W. Luo and J.J.R. Chong: no relevant disclosures.

REFERENCES

1. Krizhevsky A, Sutskever I, Hinton GE. Imagenet classification with deep convolutional neural networks. In: Pereira F, Burges CJC, Bottou L, et al. Advances in neural information processing systems. Lake Tahoe (NV): Curran Associates, Inc; 2012. p. 1097–105.
2. Friedman C, Hripcsak G. Natural language processing and its future in medicine. Acad Med 1999;74(8):890–5.
3. Pons E, Braun LM, Hunink MM, et al. Natural language processing in radiology: a systematic review. Radiology 2016;279(2):329–43.
4. Cai T, Giannopoulos AA, Yu S, et al. Natural Language Processing Technologies in Radiology Research and Clinical Applications. Radiographics 2016;36(1):176–91.
5. Chartrand G, Cheng PM, Vorontsov E, et al. Deep learning: a primer for radiologists. Radiographics 2017;37(7):2113–31.
6. Webster JJ, Kit C. Tokenization as the initial phase in NLP. In: COLING 1992 Volume 4: The 15th International Conference on Computational Linguistics. Nantes (France), August 23-28, 1992.
7. Silva C, Ribeiro B. The importance of stop word removal on recall values in text categorization. In: Proceedings of the International Joint Conference on Neural Networks. Portland (OR), July 20, 2003.
8. Balakrishnan V, Lloyd-Yemoh E. Stemming and lemmatization: a comparison of retrieval performances. In: Proceedings of SCEI Seoul Conferences. Seoul (Korea), April 10-11, 2014.
9. Plisson J, Lavrac N, Mladenic D. A rule based approach to word lemmatization. Proceedings of IS-2004. Salt Lake City (UT), May 3-5, 2004.
10. Brill E. A simple rule-based part of speech tagger. In Proceedings of the third conference on Applied natural language processing. Association for Computational Linguistics. Newark (DE), June 28-July 2, 1992.
11. Navigli R. Word sense disambiguation: A survey. ACM computing surveys (CSUR) 2009;41(2):1-69.
12. Zhang Y, Jin R, Zhou ZH. Understanding bag-of-words model: a statistical framework. International Journal of Machine Learning and Cybernetics 2010;1(1–4):43–52. https://doi.org/10.1007/s13042-010-0001-0.

13. Voorhees EM. Natural language processing and information retrieval. In: Pazienza MT, editor. International summer School on information extraction. Berlin: Springer; 1999. p. 32–48.

14. Ramos J. Using tf-idf to determine word relevance in document queries. In Proceedings of the first instructional conference on machine learning. Piscataway (NJ), December 3-8, 2003.

15. Taylor SJ, Harabagiu SM. The Role of a Deep-Learning Method for Negation Detection in Patient Cohort Identification from Electroencephalography Reports. In AMIA Annual Symposium Proceedings. American Medical Informatics Association. San Francisco (CA), November 3-7, 2018.

16. Chapman WW, Bridewell W, Hanbury P, et al. A simple algorithm for identifying negated findings and diseases in discharge summaries. J Biomed Inform 2001;34(5):301–10.

17. Mehrabi S, Krishnan A, Sohn S, et al. DEEPEN: A negation detection system for clinical text incorporating dependency relation into NegEx. J Biomed Inform 2015;54:213–9.

18. Mikolov T, Sutskever I, Chen K, et al. Distributed representations of words and phrases and their compositionality. In Advances in neural information processing systems 2013. pp. 3111–9.

19. Pennington J, Socher R, Manning C. Glove: Global vectors for word representation. In Proceedings of the 2014 conference on empirical methods in natural language processing (EMNLP). Doha (Qatar), October 25-29, 2014.

20. Banerjee I, Madhavan S, Goldman RE, et al. Intelligent word embeddings of free-text radiology reports. In AMIA Annual Symposium Proceedings. American Medical Informatics Association. Brussels (Belgium), October 31-November 4, 2018.

21. Kleene SC. Representation of events in nerve nets and finite automata. RAND PROJECT AIR FORCE SANTA MONICA CA; 1951.

22. Thompson K. Programming techniques: Regular expression search algorithm. Commun ACM 1968; 11(6):419–22.

23. Johnson WL, Porter JH, Ackley SI, et al. Automatic generation of efficient lexical processors using finite state techniques. Commun ACM 1968;11(12):805–13.

24. Pranckevičius T, Marcinkevičius V. Comparison of naive bayes, random forest, decision tree, support vector machines, and logistic regression classifiers for text reviews classification. Baltic J Mod Comput 2017;5(2):221–32.

25. LeCun Y, Bengio Y, Hinton G. Deep learning. Nature 2015;521(7553):436–44.

26. LeCun Y, Haffner P, Bottou L, et al. Object recognition with gradient-based learning. In: Forsyth DA, Mundy JL, di Gesu V, et al, editors. Shape, contour and grouping in computer vision. Berlin: Springer; 1999. p. 319–45.

27. Kim Y. Convolutional neural networks for sentence classification. In Proceedings of the 2014 conference on empirical methods in natural language processing (EMNLP). Doha (Qatar), October 25-29, 2014.

28. Elman JL. Finding structure in time. Cogn Sci 1990; 14(2):179–211.

29. Hochreiter S, Schmidhuber J. Long short-term memory. Neural Comput 1997;9(8):1735–80.

30. Lei T, Zhang Y, Wang SI, et al. Simple recurrent units for highly parallelizable recurrence. In: Proceedings of the 2018 Conference on Empirical Methods in Natural Language Processing 2018, 4470-4481.

31. Howard J, Ruder S. Universal Language Model Fine-tuning for Text Classification. In Proceedings of the 56th Annual Meeting of the Association for Computational Linguistics. Melbourne (Australia), July 15-20, 2018.

32. Devlin J, Chang MW, Lee K, et al. BERT: pre-training of deep bidirectional transformers for language understanding. Minneapolis (MN): North American Association for Computational Linguistics (NAACL); 2019.

33. Vaswani A, Shazeer N, Parmar N, et al. Attention is all you need. In: Guyon I, Luxburg UV, Bengio S, et al, editors. Advances in Neural Information Processing Systems 30. Curran Associates, Inc; 2017. p. 5998-6008.

34. You Y, Li J, Hseu J, et al. 2019. Reducing bert pre-training time from 3 days to 76 minutes. In Proceedings of the Eight International Conference on Learning Representations. Addis Ababa (Ethiopia), April 26-May 1, 2020.

35. Peters M, Neumann M, Iyyer M, et al. Deep contextualized word representations. New Orleans (LA): North American Association for Computational Linguistics (NAACL); 2018.

36. Liu Y, Ott M, Goyal N, et al. RoBERTa: A Robustly Optimized BERT Pretraining Approach. In Proceedings of the Eight International Conference on Learning Representations. Addis Ababa (Ethiopia), April 26-May 1, 2020.

37. Conneau A, Lample G. Cross-lingual Language Model Pretraining. In Advances in Neural Information Processing Systems. Vancouver (Canada), December 8-14, 2019.

38. Radford A, Wu J, Child R, et al. Language models are unsupervised multitask learners. Technical report. San Francisco (CA): OpenAI; 2019.

39. Brown AD, Marotta TR. Using machine learning for sequence-level automated MRI protocol selection in neuroradiology. J Am Med Inform Assoc 2018; 25(5):568–71.

40. Goel A, Shish G, Rasiej M, et al. Deep Learning for Comprehensive Automated Radiology Protocolling. In: SIIM 2018 Proceedings. Available at: https://cdn. ymaws.com/siim.org/resource/resmgr/siim2018/

abstracts/18ml-productivity-Goel.pdf. Accessed November 1, 2019.

41. Chen PH, Zafar H, Galperin-Aizenberg M, et al. Integrating natural language processing and machine learning algorithms to categorize oncologic response in radiology reports. J Digit Imaging 2018;31(2):178–84.

42. Wang Y, Mehrabi S, Sohn S, et al. Natural language processing of radiology reports for identification of skeletal site-specific fractures. BMC Med Inform Decis Mak 2019;19(3):73.

43. Hripcsak G, Austin JH, Alderson PO, et al. Use of natural language processing to translate clinical information from a database of 889,921 chest radiographic reports. Radiology 2002;224(1): 157–63.

44. Percha B, Nassif H, Lipson J, et al. Automatic classification of mammography reports by BI-RADS breast tissue composition class. J Am Med Inform Assoc 2012;19(5):913–6.

45. Dang PA, Kalra MK, Blake MA, et al. Natural language processing using online analytic processing for assessing recommendations in radiology reports. J Am Coll Radiol 2008;5(3):197–204.

46. Santo EC, Dunbar PJ, Sloan CE, et al. Initial effectiveness of a monitoring system to correctly identify inappropriate lack of follow-up for abdominal imaging findings of possible cancer. J Am Coll Radiol 2016;13(12):1505–8.

47. Chen MC, Ball RL, Yang L, et al. Deep learning to classify radiology free-text reports. Radiology 2017;286(3):845–52.

48. Chong J, Lee TC, Attarian A, et al. Association of lower diagnostic yield with high users of CT pulmonary angiogram. JAMA Intern Med 2018;178(3): 412–3.

49. Goff DJ, Loehfelm TW. Automated radiology report summarization using an open-source natural language processing pipeline. J Digit Imaging 2018; 31(2):185–92.

50. Bozkurt S, Alkim E, Banerjee I, et al. Automated detection of measurements and their descriptors in radiology reports using a hybrid natural language processing algorithm. J Digit Imaging 2019;32(4): 544–53.

51. Chetlen A, Artrip R, Drury B, et al. Novel use of chatbot technology to educate patients before breast biopsy. J Am Coll Radiol 2019;16(9 Pt B):1305–8.

An East Coast Perspective on Artificial Intelligence and Machine Learning: Part 1
Hemorrhagic Stroke Imaging and Triage

Rajiv Gupta, MD, PhD[a],*, Sanjith Prahas Krishnam, MBBS[b],
Pamela W. Schaefer, MD[a], Michael H. Lev, MD[c,d],
R. Gilberto Gonzalez, MD, PhD[a]

KEYWORDS

- Stroke • Hemorrhagic stroke • Intracranial hemorrhage detection
- Intracranial hemorrhage quantification • Hemorrhage expansion • Deep learning neural networks

KEY POINTS

- Artificial intelligence techniques are increasingly being used to manage patients suspected of acute ischemic or hemorrhagic stroke.
- In Part 1 of this 2-part article, we review deep learning convolutional neural networks, a specialized field of artificial intelligence, for managing hemorrhagic stroke.
- Artificial intelligence techniques for intracranial hemorrhage detection, quantification, and expansion prediction are described and illustrated with the help of examples.

INTRODUCTION

Stroke, with an annual incidence of 795,000 cases in the United States,[1] is a leading cause of disability in the United States and the second leading cause of death worldwide.[2] From an etiologic standpoint, stroke refers to 2 distinct disease entities: 87% of all strokes are ischemic in origin and the remaining are hemorrhagic strokes, with intracerebral hemorrhage (ICH) and subarachnoid hemorrhage accounting for 10% and 3% of the cases, respectively.[1,3] One-third of ischemic strokes are due to large vessel occlusion.[4]

The first goal of imaging in stroke is to differentiate among ischemic strokes, hemorrhagic strokes, and stroke mimics. For hemorrhagic strokes, noncontrast computed tomography (CT) scanning is primarily used to establish the presence of hemorrhage. In most stroke centers, noncontrast CT scanning is generally followed by a contrast-enhanced CT angiogram (CTA) with delayed or multiphase CTA image acquisition. These later images can be used to determine the etiology of the hemorrhagic stroke, for example, for elucidating any underlying arteriovenous malformation or hemorrhagic metastatic lesion. Delayed images may also help if a spot sign is present, predictive of hematoma expansion.[5]

The urgency in stroke evaluation and treatment, captured by the phrase "Time is brain," is one of the reasons that artificial intelligence (AI) and machine learning are likely to play an important role

[a] Department of Radiology, Division of Neuroradiology, Massachusetts General Hospital, Harvard Medical School, Room: GRB-273A, 55 Fruit Street, Boston, MA 02114, USA; [b] Department of Neurology, University of Alabama at Birmingham, SC 350, 1720 2nd Avenue South, Birmingham, AL 35294, USA; [c] Department of Radiology, Division of Emergency Radiology, Massachusetts General Hospital, Harvard Medical School, Room: GRB-273A, 55 Fruit Street, Boston, MA 02114, USA; [d] Department of Radiology, Division of Neuroradiology, Massachusetts General Hospital, Room: GRB-273A, 55 Fruit Street, Boston, MA 02114, USA
* Corresponding author.
E-mail address: Rgupta1@mgh.harvard.edu

Neuroimag Clin N Am 30 (2020) 459–466
https://doi.org/10.1016/j.nic.2020.07.005
1052-5149/20/© 2020 Elsevier Inc. All rights reserved.

neuroimaging.theclinics.com

in stroke neuroimaging. Automated segmentation algorithms and subsequent quantitative assessments enable timely diagnosis and treatment of strokes. AI-based methods also assist with prognostication and outcome prediction. Finally, AI-based methods can address the large geographic mismatch that is prevalent in many parts of the world: most strokes occur in suburban or rural communities and most stroke centers are located in urban areas.

In this article, we explore the usefulness of AI in the management of hemorrhagic stroke. Ischemic stroke is covered in a separate chapter. Our coverage is focused on neuroimaging and how AI can be used for the efficient, automated triage of hemorrhagic stroke. AI can be used for hemorrhage detection, segmentation, quantitation, and prediction of expansion risk.

AUTOMATIC DETECTION OF HEMORRHAGIC STROKE

The presenting clinical symptoms of acute stroke can be nonspecific and neuroimaging is often used to differentiate among ischemic stroke, hemorrhagic stroke, and stroke mimics. This distinction is paramount very early in the course of disease management because the clinical pathways are very different for these 3 entities. Typically, a noncontrast CT scan is the initial modality of choice because it has a high sensitivity for the identification of acute hemorrhage, a condition one has to definitively exclude before administering intravenous tissue plasminogen activator. Although MR imaging sequences (eg, susceptibility-weighted or gradient echo images) are equally sensitive, the limited availability of MR imaging scanners, long image acquisition times, high cost, implanted hardware, and issues with patient tolerance may limit the use of MR imaging in acute stroke imaging.[6,7]

AI algorithms can automatically detect and segment intracranial hemorrhage on noncontrast CT images. In the long term, such functionality could be useful in resource-constrained settings where a neuroradiologist is not immediately available to review images. Even when a neuroradiologic review is available, such functionality may be used to manage and prioritize the reading queue in a busy emergency department.

Multiple companies have developed automated, AI based programs for automatic hemorrhage detection in noncontrast head CT scans. A partial list of these companies includes: Accipiolx (MaxQ-AI Ltd., Tel Aviv, Israel), Aidoc Briefcase ICH (Aidoc Medical, Ltd., New York, NY), CuraRad-ICH (CuraCloud Corporation, Seattle, WA),

HealthICH (Zebra Medical Vision Ltd., Shefayim, Israel), RAPID ICH (Rapid.ai, iSchemaView, Menlo Park, CA), Viz ICH (Viz.ai Inc., San Francisco, CA). We review some recent attempts at AI-based ICH detectors where details of the AI approach have been published.

Arbabshirani and colleagues[8] (2018) described a fully 3-dimensional deep learning architecture for identification of ICH on CT scans. The proposed architecture had 5 convolutional layers and 2 fully connected layers aside from the normalization and max-pooling layers. Stochastic gradient descent was used to train the proposed network. A total of 46,583 noncontrast CT scans acquired were used for training, cross-validation, and testing. All the CT scans used in this exercise came from 17 different scanners located in different facilities and imaging centers. The scans were from 4 different manufacturers and represented a heterogeneous database of scanners, vendors, and scan protocols. **Fig. 1** shows the overall schematic of the convolutional neural network (CNN) architecture that was used for ICH detection.

The area under the receiver operating characteristic curve for predicting the presence or absence of ICH was 0.846 (95% confidence interval [CI], 0.837–0.856). The overall specificity and sensitivity were 0.800 (95% CI, 0.790–0.809) and 0.730 (95% CI, 0.713–0.748), respectively, with a false-positive rate of 20% chosen as an operating point.

It is fair to say that the performance of this CNN model is far from that of a trained radiologist. However, such a performance is adequate for prioritizing radiology workflow and reading lists. The authors tested this hypothesis by prospectively implementing the algorithm for real-time management of radiology worklists over a 3-month period. The system was used to prioritize "routine" outpatient head CT scans as "stat" scans if ICH was detected.

During the evaluation time period, 347 routine head CT scans were processed by the algorithm with an accuracy of 84% (95% CI, 78%–87%), sensitivity of 70% (95% CI, 58%–78%), and specificity of 87% (95% CI, 82%–91%). Of 347 scans on the work list, 94 (26%) were upgraded from routine to stat status. The interpreting radiologist judged 60 of the 94 upstaged scans as having an ICH (positive predictive value of 64%). The algorithm decreased the median time to diagnosis from 512 minutes to 19 minutes by prioritizing routine scans as stat scans. This demonstrates the usefulness of machine learning in radiology workflow optimization.

Lee and colleagues[9] (2018) developed a deep learning CNN to detect acute intracranial

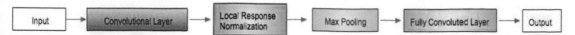

Fig. 1. Schematic depiction of the CNN architecture used by Arbabshirani and colleagues[8] (2018) for identification of ICH on CT scans. It contains 5 convolutional layers and 2 fully connected layers. (*Adapted from* Arbabshirani MR, Fornwalt BK, Mongelluzzo GJ, et al. Advanced machine learning in action: identification of intracranial hemorrhage on computed tomography scans of the head with clinical workflow integration. Npj Digit Med. 2018;1(1):1-7. https://doi.org/10.1038/s41746-017-0015-z; used with permission.)

hemorrhage in noncontrast head CT scans. The system was also trained to classify the ICH into the 5 subtypes. The authors used a preprocessing pipeline, multiple ImageNet pretrained deep CNNs, an atlas creation module, and a prediction-basis selection module. Although the training and validation datasets consisted of only 904 cases, the skewed distribution of training data was counteracted with a preprocessing pipeline and network optimization techniques. This process included an output that predicts the probability of any type of ICH, additional costs for misclassification of positive instances, a multi-window conversion, and slice interpolation. Four deep CNNs—namely, VGG167, ResNet-508, Inception-v39, and Inception-ResNet-v210— were used to build the model.

The authors tested the model on a retrospective and a prospective dataset consisting of a combination of different types of ICH with testing being carried out at the case level rather than slice level. For ICH detection the model achieved an area under the receiver operating characteristic curve of 0.99 (95% CI, 0.982–0.999) on the retrospective test set and an area under the receiver operating characteristic curve of 0.96 (95% CI, 0.927–0.986) on the prospective test set. For the retrospective test set, the sensitivity and specificity for ICH detection were 98.0% (95% CI, 95.3%–100%) and 95.0% (95% CI, 90.7%–99.3%), respectively. For the prospective test set, the sensitivity was 92.4% (95% CI, 86.6%–98.2%) and the specificity was 94.9% (95% CI, 90.9%–98.9%). The performance of the model was comparable to radiologists on the retrospective test set, but the sensitivity of the model was superior to radiologists in the case of the prospective test set. For the ICH classification, the model demonstrated area under the receiver operating characteristic curve values between 0.92 (epidural hemorrhage) to 0.98 (intraparenchymal hemorrhage) in the retrospective set and between 0.88 (subdural hematoma) and 0.97 (intraventricular hemorrhage) in the prospective test set.

In addition to the identification and classification of ICH, the CNN also generated attention maps to localize bleeding points. Overall, 78.1% of the

bleeding points annotated by the neuroradiologists overlapped with the attention maps. To make model decisions more understandable to the users, the authors also developed an atlas of the relevant features of each subtype of ICH from the training dataset. The model then provided the prediction basis for a given case by retrieving images from the training datasets relevant to the features from the atlas. The agreement between 3 independent neuroradiologists and the algorithm for selecting morphologically similar prediction basis images was 93% to 95%.

Chilamkurthy and colleagues[10] (2018) reported a deep learning algorithm for the detection of critical findings in head CT scans to serve as an automated head CT scan triage system. In addition to detecting the same 5 subtypes of ICH as Lee and colleagues,[9] the trained algorithm also detected mass effect, midline shift, and calvarial fractures. The model was trained and validated with 313,318 head CT scans from 20 different centers in India reflecting a heterogeneous dataset. The authors also used an additional validation dataset sourced from a center distinct from those that provided the training dataset. The algorithm consistently achieved an area under the receiver operating characteristic curve greater than 0.9 for both validation datasets in identifying ICH and its subtypes.

HEMORRHAGE SEGMENTATION AND QUANTITATION

The volume of ICH is the single most important factor in predicting the mortality in a patient with hemorrhagic stroke. Multiple AI-based algorithms have been developed to segment and quantitate ICH volume. For illustrative purposes, we describe one such attempt from our group.

Coorens and colleagues[11] (2019) developed an algorithm based on CNNs using the U-Net architecture combined with a masked loss function to automatically detect and segment ICH in noncontrast CT images. **Fig. 2** shows the CNN architecture used in this research prototype.

In this prototype system, 107 CT scans were used for training, testing, and validation of the algorithm. The model could detect hemorrhage

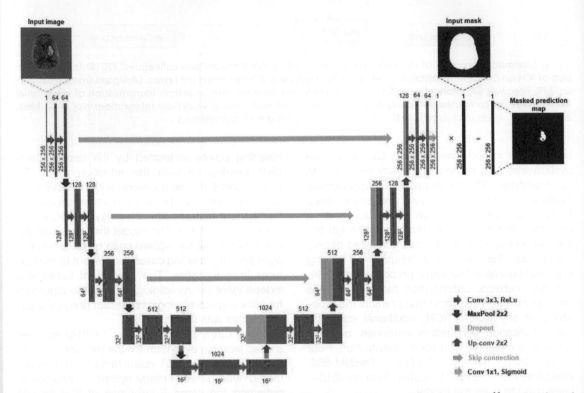

Fig. 2. Schematic illustration of the CNN architecture used to segment intracerebral hematomas.[11] A U-Net based on the work of Ronneberger and colleagues (2019)[12] was combined with a masked loss function. The output of the final convolutional layer is multiplied with the mask of the input image. (*Adapted from* Ronneberger O, Fischer P, Brox T. U-Net: Convolutional Networks for Biomedical Image Segmentation. In: Navab N, Hornegger J, Wells WM, Frangi AF, eds. Medical Image Computing and Computer-Assisted Intervention – MICCAI 2015. Lecture Notes in Computer Science. Springer International Publishing; 2015:234-241. https://doi.org/10.1007/978-3-319-24574-4_28 used with permission.)

with a sensitivity and specificity of 77% and 96.2%, respectively. When automatic segmentation was compared with manual segmentation, the model was very accurate on the segmentation task, as demonstrated by multiple metrics: the system achieved a median Dice coefficient of 75.9%, a Hausdorff distance (HD) of 2.65 pixels, a correlation coefficient of 0.97 between ICH volumes and predicted volumes, a very low bias of 0.89 mL, and limits of agreement between 4.75 mL and 6.93 mL. Although the results are promising, the low sensitivity when manual segmentation was compared with automatic segmentation prevented its immediate use in clinical practice. **Fig. 3** illustrates some results obtained from the proposed network.

PREDICTION OF HEMORRHAGE EXPANSION

ICH[13] carries a high mortality rate of approximately 40%.[14] Predictors of outcome after ICH include the volume of ICH, Glasgow coma scale score, presence of intraventricular blood, and age,

among others. Significant hematoma expansion has been reported in at least 38% of patients after onset[15] and in up to 50% of patients who are on anticoagulation.[16] The typical time course for hematoma expansion is up to 9 hours in noncoagulopathic ICH and up to 24 hours in coagulopathic ICH.[14] It is well-established that hematoma expansion in the early hours post ictus is strongly associated with a poor outcome.[14] As such, it is one of the most important independent predictors of neurologic deterioration, functional outcome, and mortality after ICH.[17] Therefore, AI-based programs that can identify patients who are at risk for hematoma expansion may help to direct management. In particular, such programs can play a pivotal role in selecting candidates for early targeted medical or surgical interventions.[5]

Hematoma expansion can potentially lead to midline shift, hydrocephalus, mass effect, and increased intracranial pressure. Such complications are associated with increased mortality and worse functional and neurologic outcomes. The risk of long-term disability increases by 7% for

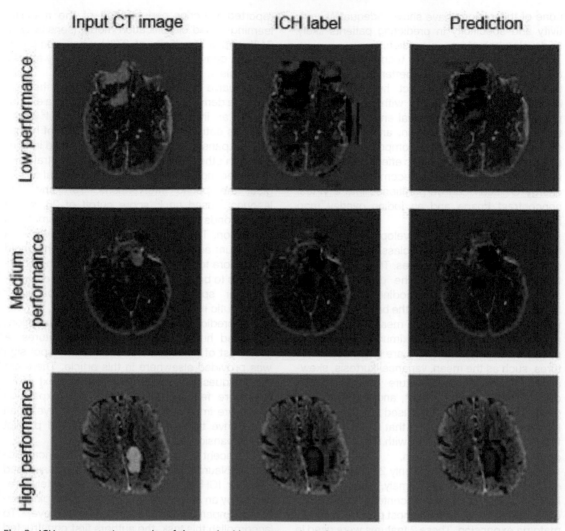

Fig. 3. ICH segmentation results of the masked loss U-Net. The left column depicts the virtual noncontrast images as presented to the U-Net. The corresponding ICH label images are shown in the middle column, and the predicted segmentation results are displayed on the right. From top to bottom, a low performing prediction (Dice = 75.3%, HD = 8.31), a medium prediction (Dice = 76.3%, HD = 2.65) and a good prediction (Dice = 97.6%, HD = 2.00) are shown. (*Courtesy of* N. Coorens, University of Twente, Enschede, the Netherlands.)

every 1 mm of hematoma expansion.[17] Nearly 28% to 38% of patients with ICH undergoing head CT scans within 3 hours of onset report hematoma expansion.[15,17]

CTA has been extensively used to assess the risk of hematoma expansion. Several radiologic parameters in both noncontrast CT and CTA imaging have been used for the evaluation of ICH expansion. In the literature, there are multiple imaging markers that have been found to be associated with ICH expansion. These radiologic markers include initial hematoma volume,[18,19] patterns of attenuation within the hematoma on CT images,[20,21] and the spot sign on CTA.[22] The spot sign—that is, the presence of foci of

hyperintensities within the hematoma on a delayed CTA that are believed to represent areas of active contrast extravasation—is an independent risk factor for hematoma expansion with a sensitivity of 50% to 60% and specificity of 80% to 90%.[22–24] As such, the spot sign is highly specific for hematoma expansion.[25] However, it has a relatively low sensitivity.[26,27]

The radiologic literature is full of other correlative signs, such as hematoma location, descriptive markers such as shape and density, hemorrhagic time course, multifocality of bleeding, the island sign,[28] the satellite sign,[29] the black hole sign,[30] the blend sign,[31] the swirl sign,[32] margin irregularity,[33] and hematoma hypodensities.[23] Overall, none of these signs have shown adequate sensitivity and specificity in predicting patients likely to develop hematoma expansion.

Advanced neuroradiology techniques such as dual energy CT scans may better optimize radiologic signs that can detect hemorrhage and improve its characterization with respect to the probability of expansion. Dual energy CTA helps to identify hemorrhage, brain, and contrast medium through 3 material decomposition using the principles of the photoelectric effect and Compton scattering. Using material decomposition, a dual energy CT scan can be partitioned into a virtual noncontrast image and an iodine overlay map image.

Tan and colleagues[34] developed an machine learning-based naïve Bayes classifier using quantitative dual energy CT features. The following features were derived from the dual energy CT angiography and explored: iodine content in the hematoma, iodine content in the brightest spot, total iodine content in all spots, mean iodine content per voxel in all spots, and maximum iodine content per voxel in all spots. There are many other features, such as the mean, variance, kurtosis, skewness, texture entropy, texture energy, texture dissimilarity, texture contrast, and texture homogeneity, that could also be used in the classifier. However, the authors found that these other features were highly correlated with these 5 features derived from the iodine maps.

After a detailed analysis, only 2 of these 5 dual energy CT parameters—namely, iodine content in the hematoma and iodine content in the brightest spot—were found to be most predictive for hematoma expansion. These 2 features were used in a naïve Bayes classifier for differentiating between the expanders and nonexpanders. The authors defined a new score, called the I^2 score, that combines these 2 features in a single metric. They reported superior performance of the machine learning-based classification model (sensitivity of 71% and a specificity of 97%) when compared with the conventional spot sign as read by trained radiologists.

The naïve Bayes classification allows the prospective derivation of the risk of hematoma expansion at an individual level because the I^2 score stratifies patients according to their risk of hematoma expansion. The I^2 score can be used in concert with other known risk factors when stratifying and selecting patients for possible medical or surgical therapeutic interventions. Tan and colleagues[34] used an I^2 score cutoff of 26, which corresponds with a 30% probability of hematoma expansion. The risk of expansion, however, is a continuum and one may use a different threshold on I^2 score for separating expanders from nonexpanders to better match the need for higher sensitivity or specificity required by a particular therapeutic intervention.

The prediction of ICH expansion has traditionally used human-derived radiologic features. A partial list of these features such as the spot sign was provided elsewhere in this article. There are natural questions that arise in the context of AI. Are there features that predict ICH expansion which are imperceptible to the human eye? Can one derive these features using AI and predict ICH expansion with higher accuracy?

In a recent paper presented at the American Society of Neuroradiology (2020), Lipman[35] assessed whether ICH expansion can be accurately predicted by an AI system that leverages imaging features imperceptible to the human eye. To accomplish this task, the authors first constructed an optimal CNN architecture by searching the space of hyperparameters that define a CNN architecture using Bayesian optimization and Gaussian processes. They then trained the optimal

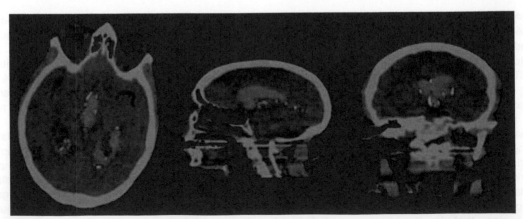

Fig. 4. Saliency map of an expander projected on the virtual noncontrast images derived from dual energy CT.

CNN using a relatively modest-sized training set. They showed that it is possible to derive a task-specific CNN using Bayesian optimization that achieves 82.7% accuracy, 66.7% sensitivity, 75% precision, and 90.0% specificity at dual-energy CT scans of the brain.

This paper describes a radical departure from the usual paradigm of taking a given CNN architecture and training it until the improvement in model performance reaches a plateau. It shows that automatic architecture optimization may help to select an optimal, task-specific AI architecture. For ICH expansion prediction, this paradigm can provide an accuracy and specificity similar to the best performing algorithms based on human-derived radiologic assessment. It also illustrates that there are radiographic features of an expanding hematoma that are currently unknown to radiologists, as demonstrated by the saliency maps that show regions where the CNN is gleaning information about hematoma expansion. To date, all imaging features, such as hematoma texture, spot sign, and other, have typically used features that reside in the middle of the hematoma. The saliency map of an expanding hematoma is shown in **Fig. 4**. As can be seen, **Fig. 4** shows that an AI-based system is leveraging information at the edges of the hematoma and not in the middle.

SUMMARY

AI is playing an increasing role in the management of hemorrhagic stroke. Multiple articles have discussed detection, segmentation, and quantitation of hemorrhage in the setting of stroke. Work is also on going in hematoma expansion prediction. One can also envision in future automated programs that can guide triage in terms of interventions such as hematoma evacuation. Similarly, it may be possible to train a CNN and predict patient outcomes using imaging and clinical features. It is safe to say that in future, AI will play a key role in guiding and informing both neuroimaging and subsequent triage. Future applications and challenges are discussed in the article on ischemic stroke.

DISCLOSURE

The authors have nothing to disclose.

REFERENCES

1. Benjamin EJ, Blaha MJ, Chiuve SE, et al. Heart disease and stroke statistics-2017 update: a report from the American Heart Association. Circulation 2017;135(10):e146–603.
2. Writing Group Members, Mozaffarian D, Benjamin EJ, et al. Heart disease and stroke statistics-2016 update: a report from the American Heart Association. Circulation 2016;133(4):e38–360.
3. Gebel JM, Broderick JP. Intracerebral hemorrhage. Neurol Clin 2000;18(2):419–38.
4. Malhotra K, Gornbein J, Saver JL. Ischemic strokes due to large-vessel occlusions contribute disproportionately to stroke-related dependence and death: a review. Front Neurol 2017;8:651.
5. Romero JM, Brouwers HB, Lu J, et al. Prospective validation of the computed tomographic angiography spot sign score for intracerebral hemorrhage. Stroke 2013;44(11):3097–102.
6. Fiebach Jochen B, Schellinger Peter D, Achim G, et al. Stroke magnetic resonance imaging is accurate in hyperacute intracerebral hemorrhage. Stroke 2004;35(2):502–6.
7. Chalela JA, Kidwell CS, Nentwich LM, et al. Magnetic resonance imaging and computed tomography in emergency assessment of patients with suspected acute stroke: a prospective comparison. Lancet Lond Engl 2007;369(9558):293–8.
8. Arbabshirani MR, Fornwalt BK, Mongelluzzo GJ, et al. Advanced machine learning in action: identification of intracranial hemorrhage on computed tomography scans of the head with clinical workflow integration. NPJ Digit Med 2018;1(1):1–7.
9. Lee H, Yune S, Mansouri M, et al. An explainable deep-learning algorithm for the detection of acute intracranial haemorrhage from small datasets. Nat Biomed Eng 2019;3(3):173–82.
10. Chilamkurthy S, Ghosh R, Tanamala S, et al. Deep learning algorithms for detection of critical findings in head CT scans: a retrospective study. Lancet Lond Engl 2018;392(10162):2388–96.
11. Coorens N, Krishnam SP, Paramhans S, et al. Segmentation on non-contrast computed tomography scans using a masked-loss U-Net. Enschede (the Netherlands): University of Twente; 2019.
12. Ronneberger O, Fischer P, Brox T. U-Net: Convolutional Networks for Biomedical Image Segmentation. In: Navab N, Hornegger J, Wells W, et al, editors. Medical Image Computing and Computer-Assisted Intervention – MICCAI 2015. MICCAI 2015. Lecture Notes in Computer Science, vol 9351. Springer, Cham. https://doi.org/10.1007/978-3-319-24574-4_28.
13. Feigin VL, Lawes CMM, Bennett DA, et al. Worldwide stroke incidence and early case fatality reported in 56 population-based studies: a systematic review. Lancet Neurol 2009;8(4):355–69.
14. Demchuk AM, Dowlatshahi D, Rodriguez-Luna D, et al. Prediction of haematoma growth and outcome in patients with intracerebral haemorrhage using the CT-angiography spot sign (PREDICT): a prospective observational study. Lancet Neurol 2012;11(4):307–14.
15. Brott T, Broderick J, Kothari R, et al. Early hemorrhage growth in patients with intracerebral hemorrhage. Stroke 1997;28(1):1–5.

16. Flibotte JJ, Hagan N, O'Donnell J, et al. Warfarin, hematoma expansion, and outcome of intracerebral hemorrhage. Neurology 2004;63(6):1059–64.

17. Davis SM, Broderick J, Hennerici M, et al. Hematoma growth is a determinant of mortality and poor outcome after intracerebral hemorrhage. Neurology 2006;66(8):1175–81.

18. Takeda R, Ogura T, Ooigawa H, et al. A practical prediction model for early hematoma expansion in spontaneous deep ganglionic intracerebral hemorrhage. Clin Neurol Neurosurg 2013;115(7):1028–31.

19. Brouwers HB, Chang Y, Falcone GJ, et al. Predicting hematoma expansion after primary intracerebral hemorrhage. JAMA Neurol 2014;71(2):158–64.

20. Barras CD, Tress BM, Christensen S, et al. Quantitative CT densitometry for predicting intracerebral hemorrhage growth. Am J Neuroradiol 2013;34(6):1139–44.

21. Boulouis G, Morotti A, Charidimou A, et al. Noncontrast computed tomography markers of intracerebral hemorrhage expansion. Stroke 2017;48(4):1120–5.

22. Delgado Almandoz JE, Yoo AJ, Stone MJ, et al. Systematic characterization of the computed tomography angiography spot sign in primary intracerebral hemorrhage identifies patients at highest risk for hematoma expansion. Stroke J Cereb Circ 2009;40(9):2994–3000.

23. Boulouis G, Morotti A, Brouwers HB, et al. Association Between Hypodensities Detected by Computed Tomography and Hematoma Expansion in Patients With Intracerebral Hemorrhage. JAMA Neurol 2016;73(8):961–8.

24. Wada R, Aviv RI, Fox AJ, et al. CT angiography "spot sign" predicts hematoma expansion in acute intracerebral hemorrhage. Stroke 2007;38(4):1257–62.

25. Phan CM, Yoo AJ, Hirsch JA, et al. Differentiation of hemorrhage from iodinated contrast in different intracranial compartments using dual-energy head CT. AJNR Am J Neuroradiol 2012;33(6):1088–94.

26. Giudice AD, D'Amico D, Sobesky J, et al. Accuracy of the spot sign on computed tomography angiography as a predictor of haematoma enlargement after acute spontaneous intracerebral haemorrhage: a systematic review. Cerebrovasc Dis 2014;37(4):268–76.

27. Du F-Z, Jiang R, Gu M, et al. The accuracy of spot sign in predicting hematoma expansion after intracerebral hemorrhage: a systematic review and meta-analysis. PLoS One 2014;9(12):e115777.

28. Li Q, Liu Q-J, Yang W-S, et al. Island sign: an imaging predictor for early hematoma expansion and poor outcome in patients with intracerebral hemorrhage. Stroke 2017;48(11):3019–25.

29. Yu Z, Zheng J, Ali H, et al. Significance of satellite sign and spot sign in predicting hematoma expansion in spontaneous intracerebral hemorrhage. Clin Neurol Neurosurg 2017;162:67–71.

30. Yu Z, Zheng J, Ma L, et al. The predictive accuracy of the black hole sign and the spot sign for hematoma expansion in patients with spontaneous intracerebral hemorrhage. Neurol Sci 2017;38(9):1591–7.

31. Li Q, Yang W-S, Wang X-C, et al. Blend sign predicts poor outcome in patients with intracerebral hemorrhage. PLoS One 2017;12(8):e0183082.

32. Selariu E, Zia E, Brizzi M, et al. Swirl sign in intracerebral haemorrhage: definition, prevalence, reliability and prognostic value. BMC Neurol 2012;12(1):109.

33. Blacquiere D, Demchuk AM, Al-Hazzaa M, et al. Intracerebral hematoma morphologic appearance on noncontrast computed tomography predicts significant hematoma expansion. Stroke 2015;46(11):3111–6.

34. Tan CO, Lam S, Kuppens D, et al. Spot and diffuse signs: quantitative markers of intracranial hematoma expansion at dual-energy CT. Radiology 2018;290(1):179–86.

35. Lipman K. Deep learning-based prediction of intracerebral hemorrhage expansion with Dual-Energy Computed Tomography. Oral Presentation presented at the: ASNR 2020, 58th Annual Meeting; Las Vegas, NV, June 30, 2020.

An East Coast Perspective on Artificial Intelligence and Machine Learning
Part 2: Ischemic Stroke Imaging and Triage

Rajiv Gupta, MD, PhD[a],*, Sanjith Prahas Krishnam, MBBS[b],
Pamela W. Schaefer, MD[a], Michael H. Lev, MD[c,d],
R. Gilberto Gonzalez, MD, PhD[a]

KEYWORDS

- Stroke • Ischemic stroke • Ischemic stroke detection • Stroke segmentation
- Deep learning neural networks

KEY POINTS

- In Part 2 of this 2-part review, we review artificial intelligence techniques, specifically, deep learning convolutional neural networks, for managing ischemic stroke.
- Artificial intelligence techniques may be used to detect and localize acute ischemic stroke on early computed tomography images and segment diffusion-weighted MR images to automatically measure the size of the infarct.
- Artificial intelligence techniques may be used to automatically detect large vessel occlusion on a computed tomography angiogram and to process computed tomography perfusion images for detection of ischemic core and penumbra.
- This article describes artificial intelligence techniques for solving these problems and illustrates them with the help of examples.

INTRODUCTION

One-third of all strokes are ischemic strokes caused by large vessel occlusions (LVOs). LVOs are responsible for 90% of mortality in ischemic strokes, with survivors suffering severe neurologic disability.[1] Once hemorrhage is excluded and the diagnosis of ischemic stroke is established, further management is focused on whether it is advisable to reestablish blood flow to the ischemic territory, and how that should be accomplished.

Ischemic stroke care has undergone monumental changes over the past 2 decades. In 1995 the National Institute of Neurologic Disorders and Stroke conducted the tissue plasminogen activator (tPA) trial that showed improved outcomes with tPA administration within 3 hours. In 2008, the therapeutic window for tPA administration was extended from 3.0 hours to 4.5 hours.[2] Currently, tPA is the only intravenous (IV) treatment for ischemic or thrombotic stroke approved by the US Food and Drug Administration. Despite

[a] Department of Radiology, Division of Neuroradiology, Massachusetts General Hospital, Harvard Medical School, Room: GRB-273A, 55 Fruit Street, Boston, MA 02114, USA; [b] Department of Neurology, University of Alabama at Birmingham, SC 350, 1720 2nd Avenue South, Birmingham, AL 35294, USA; [c] Department of Radiology, Division of Emergency Radiology, Massachusetts General Hospital, Harvard Medical School, Boston, MA, USA; [d] Department of Radiology, Division of Neuroradiology, Massachusetts General Hospital, Room: GRB-273A, 55 Fruit Street, Boston, MA 02114, USA
* Corresponding author.
E-mail address: Rgupta1@mgh.harvard.edu

Neuroimag Clin N Am 30 (2020) 467–478
https://doi.org/10.1016/j.nic.2020.08.002

extensive literature that establishes the benefits of IV tPA administration in the appropriate time window, most patients do not reach an emergency room within the mandated time window of 4.5 hours. Multiple other compounds such as desmoteplase and tenecteplase are in clinical trials for determining their efficacy with a view to possibly lengthening the IV treatment window.[1,3–5]

In 2015, the results from 5 clinical trials—MR CLEAN, ESCAPE, REVESCAT, EXTEND IA, and SWIFT-PRIME—demonstrated the benefit of endovascular mechanical thrombectomy over best medical therapy (including IV-tPA when appropriate) if performed within 6 hours of symptom onset of ischemic stroke.[6–10] In late 2017 and early 2018, respectively, the DAWN and DEFUSE 3 trials reported the benefit of endovascular mechanical thrombectomy up to 24 hours from the symptom onset in the setting of proximal LVO. In all these trials, neuroimaging formed the basis for patient selection.[11,12]

For ischemic stroke, the first tasks are to rule out hemorrhage, identify the presence and site of occlusion or stenosis, and determine the size of the infarct core using noninvasive means. Exclusion of hemorrhage on a head computed tomography (CT), identification of anterior circulation LVO on CT angiography (CTA) and exclusion of a large, well-established infarct core on CT, CTA, CT perfusion (CTP) or diffusion-weighted imaging (DWI) are the main triage modalities that are used for patient selection for revascularization therapy.[13]

In certain situations, especially in cases of anterior circulation strokes where there is a large mismatch between infarct core and ischemic penumbra, it has been shown that appropriately selected patients benefit from mechanical thrombectomy. DAWN and DEFUSE 3 trials proved a strong benefit of endovascular therapy in patients with anterior circulation LVOs, even in the delayed time window extending up to 24 hours after symptom onset.[11,12] Thus, further management of ischemic strokes requires additional imaging studies to identify the site of arterial occlusion, the volume of the infarcted tissue, and the volume of the ischemic penumbra that defines the tissue at risk.

In general, advances in neuroimaging have been coupled with advancements in stroke care and form the basis for several key decisions in treatment triage. The use of artificial intelligence (AI) and machine learning may further propel this partnership and usher a new era in automated stroke triage. In this article, we explore the usefulness of AI in the management of ischemic stroke and how AI could be used for decision making and efficient, automated triage.

The following questions, which can be addressed by AI, are pertinent to ischemic stroke management. We discuss them in the sections that follow.

1. Can one detect and localize acute ischemic stroke on early CT images?
2. Can we segment diffusion-weighted MR images and automatically measure the size of the infarct?
3. Can we automatically detect LVOs on a CT angiogram?
4. Can one process CTP images using AI techniques to automatically detect the core and penumbra of an acute ischemic stroke?

INFARCT LOCALIZATION ON COMPUTED TOMOGRAPHY SCANS

Although MR imaging is highly sensitive and accurate for estimation of infarct volume, the widespread use of MR imaging in acute stroke imaging is constrained by its limited availability, workflow related limitations, and long scan times. Quantification of infarct on CT scans would be ideal from a workflow point of view.

Multiple companies are developing AI-based software for processing CT stroke images. These companies include ContaCT (Viz.ai, Inc., San Francisco, CA), CT CoPilot (ZepMed, LLC, San Diego, CA), VisCTP (Viz.ai, Inc.), and VitreaCT (Vital Images, Inc., Minnetonka, MN). The holy grail of stroke assessment on CT scans is to detect and delineate infarcted territory on single or dual-energy noncontrast head CT scans. This problem is difficult and it is unclear if noncontrast CT scans have enough information in them for this task.

Large databases with head CT scans and matching MR imaging scans performed in close temporal proximity are available. One way to develop a CT scan-based stroke detector would be to train a convolutional neural network (CNN) using a noncontrast CT scan as input and the gold standard DWI image as the expected output. One can take this approach one step further and use a combination of noncontrast CT scan, CTA, and delayed CTA scans that have been cross-registered with each other as the input for training. When such a triple-phase CT scan is used, more information about the blood perfusion in the brain parenchyma is available, possibly resulting in a more accurate quantification of the infarct core.

One can further enrich the information mix by using a dual-energy CT (DECT) scan instead of a single energy CT. DECT enables quantification of iodine in DECTA, a feature that may carry information about the perfusion status of the tissue at risk.

DECT uses scanning at 2 different energies to decompose tissue into 3 different materials based on differences in contribution of photoelectric effect and Compton scattering to X-ray attenuation.[14,15] Using 3-material decomposition, DECTA source volumes can be decomposed into virtual noncontrast images and iodine only maps. Virtual noncontrast images are similar to conventional noncontrast CT scan and can reliably capture any hemorrhage. If the arterial phase and delayed phase DECTAs are acquired, as is the case at many institutions, iodine overlay images are available at 2 different time points. Iodine only map images, therefore, may provide valuable information about the distribution of blood and the presence of collaterals in nonaffected and ischemic brain tissues.

Metselaar and colleagues[16] (2019) used a conditional Generative Adversarial Network framework to generate synthetic DWI images from triple-phase CT data. A combination of noncontrast CT scan, early and delayed phase CTA images from 293 patients (184 single energy CT and 109 DECT) along with their corresponding DWI images were used to train, test, and validate the algorithm.

Fig. 1 schematically shows a CNN that was trained using triple-phase CT data and the corresponding DWI data to provide the ground truth for the infarct core. In this figure, X_0 denotes a registered triple-phase CT image consisting of a noncontrast CT scan, a CTA, and a delayed CTA, whereas X_L denotes the labeled output showing the segmented infarct in the DWI images. The network architecture, which is shown with appropriate feedforward links but without specific hyperparameters used in training, is presented only for illustrative purposes.

Fig. 2 shows an example output from the trained network. Given a triple-phase DECT dataset consisting of noncontrast CT scan, CTA, and delayed CTA, the system is able to produce realistic pseudo-DWI images. CNN accomplishes this in 2 steps. It first makes an anatomy specific pseudo-DWI image and then fuses it with a predicted

mask of the infarct. This process is illustrated elsewhere in this article (**Fig. 3**).

In **Fig. 3**, the top row shows the triphasic CT inputs to the CNN, namely, the noncontrast head CT scan, the early CTA, and the delayed CTA. The DWI image for this test case, which was not used for training, is shown in the bottom left panel. In the training set, as well as in this case, all the DWI images acquired within 45 minutes of acquiring the CT scan. In this research, we assumed that the infarct core during this time period is stable and has not substantially grown from the CT scan to the MR imaging scan. The DWI image was manually segmented to assess the boundaries of the infarct core. This segmented image is shown in the bottom middle panel and the output of the trained CNN is shown in the bottom right panel. As can be seen, the volume of the infarct core from the DWI image is very well approximated by the predicted core from the CT images.

As can be seen from this example, the trained CNN network is able to generate images that resemble the DWI images with regard to intensity and topology. However, the trained network was inconsistent in mapping the infarct from the CT information. Although major anatomic structures could be reconstructed in the pseudo- DWI images, inaccuracies in mapping the ischemic region suggest the need for further research and investigation in this promising area. This research is a work in progress and final validation results that assess the quality of CT scan-based prediction on a large test set are still awaited.

INFARCT VOLUME ESTIMATION USING MR IMAGING

Many companies are pioneering software packages for head MR imaging analysis. These software packages, some of which are already approved by the US Food and Drug Administration and/or CE marked, include cNeuro cMRI (Combinostics, Tampere, Finland), IB Neuro (Imaging Biometrics, LLC, Elm Grove, WI), Icobrain (icometrix NV, Leuven, Belgium), NeuroQuant (CorTech Labs, Inc, La Jolla, CA), QuantBrain (Quantib B.V., Rotterdam, the Netherlands), and SublteMR system for Head MR imaging Super Resolution (Subtle Medical, Inc, San Francisco, CA). Some of these packages also offer support for stroke imaging.

MR DWI are based on the measurement of the Brownian movement of the water molecules in brain tissue. Acute ischemic stroke results in cell membrane dysfunction causing cytotoxic edema and restricted diffusion of water.[17] This difference

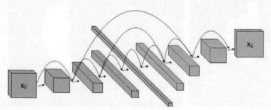

Fig. 1. A CCN for producing a DWI mask using CT scans, CTA, and delayed CTA as input. The network was trained using DWI images.

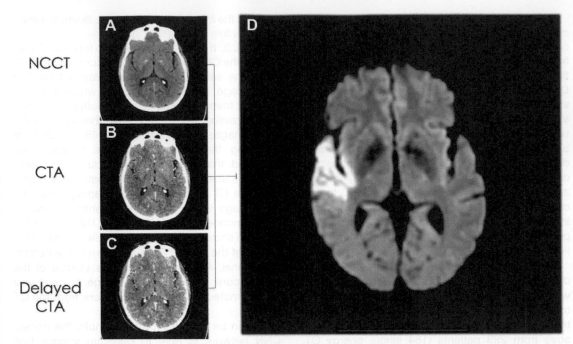

Fig. 2. A pseudo-DWI image (*right*) generated from triple-phase DECT data (*left*) by the trained CNN shown in Fig. 1.

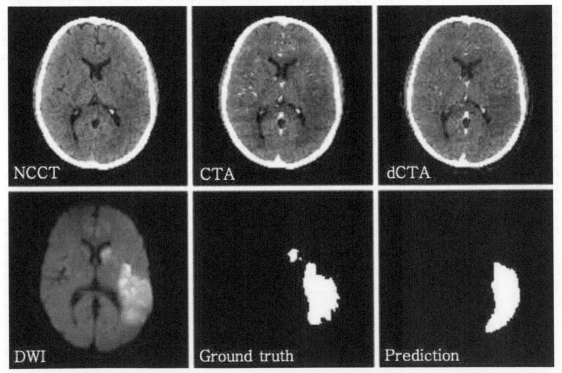

Fig. 3. Input triphasic CT scan and the corresponding DWI image for a patient with acute ischemic stroke. The ground truth volume of the infarct core from the DWI image, and predicted core from the CT images illustrate the prediction accuracy of this method.

in diffusion enables the detection of the ischemic area, which appears as a hyperintense lesion on DWI.[17] DWI in combination with apparent diffusion coefficient (ADC) maps are used to identify and segment ischemic zones while ruling out T2 shine through (which also produces a hyperintense image on DWI). DWI and ADC maps have a significantly higher signal-to-noise ratio as compared with CT images for detecting infarct. DWI can detect an infarct with a sensitivity of 74% and 94% within 3 hours and 6 hours of symptom onset, respectively.

The size of the DWI lesion can be used as a surrogate for the infarct core. Areas that are DWI bright and ADC dark are a close approximation of irreversibly injured ischemic tissue. DWI and fluid attenuated inversion recovery mismatch may also be used in the management of wake-up strokes, where the exact time of onset is sometimes unknown. In these images, the DWI map is used to label cytotoxic edema as a surrogate for the infarcted tissue; the fluid attenuated inversion recovery signal indicates the region of vasogenic edema because of hypoxia or oligemia. These considerations are factored into the decisions regarding endovascular mechanical thrombectomy.

A key task in stroke triage using MR imaging is to estimate the size of the DWI lesion. One can use the ellipsoidal rule to estimate the infarct volume. This rule requires one to first measure the 3 principal axes of the DWI lesion approximated as an ellipsoid. The infarct volume can be approximated by the product of the 3 principal axes divided by 2. Although it is quick and easy to apply, there are 2 levels of approximations in this estimate. First, the infarct shape may or may not look like an ellipsoid. Second, instead of the true volume of the ellipsoid, it is being approximated by the rule. It would be better to measure the infarct volume without these unnecessary approximations.

One can manually segment out the infarct on a DWI image. However, manual delineation of ischemic areas is a tedious and time-consuming task requiring trained radiologists for interpreting DWI while reviewing the ADC map. Deep learning algorithms can automate this process and assist physicians with automatic segmentation of lesions.

Hamelink and Gupta[18] (2019) developed a multimodal 2D CNN based on the U-Net architecture for automatic segmentation of ischemic areas using DWI and ADC images. **Fig. 4** illustrates the

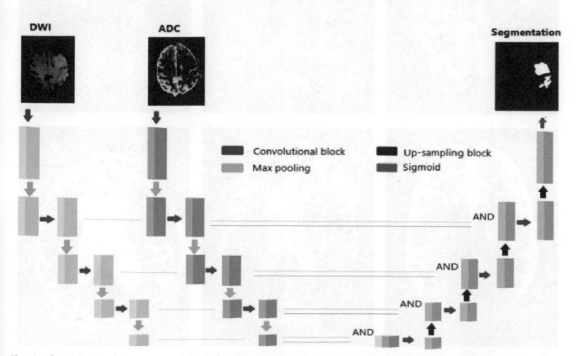

Fig. 4. The U-Net architecture used for infarct core segmentation on DWI and ADC maps. (*Adapted from* Dolz J, Ben Ai, Desrosiers C. Dense Multi-path U-Net for Ischemic Stroke Lesion Segmentation in Multiple Image Modalities. In: Crimi A., Bakas S., Kuijf H., Keyvan F., Reyes M., van Walsum T. (eds) Brainlesion: Glioma, Multiple Sclerosis, Stroke and Traumatic Brain Injuries. BrainLes 2018. Lecture Notes in Computer Science, vol 11383. Springer, Cham; with permission.)

network architecture of the proposed model. The model used 2 contracting paths, one for DWI and the other for the ADC map, followed by a late-stage modality fusion at the end of the contracting paths. This architecture enables the network to capture complex relationships between DWI and ADC maps to reject regions that represent T2 shine through. Modality fusion was achieved with an element-wise minimum operation to combine the convolved and identity feature maps in each up-convolution operation. Element-wise minimum operation acts as an AND operation, meaning that element-wise minimum lets features pass through if they are present in both DWI and ADC feature maps. Following the segmentation of the 2-dimensional input slices, the 3-dimensional volumes were reconstructed by stacking the 2-dimensional slices. Performance metrics were then calculated to assess the quality of segmentation of the original 3-dimensional volume.

The network was optimized using a generalized dice loss and achieved a Dice similarity coefficient of 0.69, a Hausdorff distance of 13 mm, and a volumetric similarity of 0.75. **Fig. 5** demonstrates some typical results from this network. The low Hausdorff distance indicates accurate segmentation of ischemic stroke lesion boundaries, which is crucial to estimating the size of the penumbra. A volumetric similarity of 0.75 indicates that the network underestimates the penumbra, which may potentially affect clinical decision making and have adverse consequences. Another limitation is that the network processes 2-dimensional slices independently and 3-dimensional images may provide additional contextual information, which may increase the segmentation accuracy.

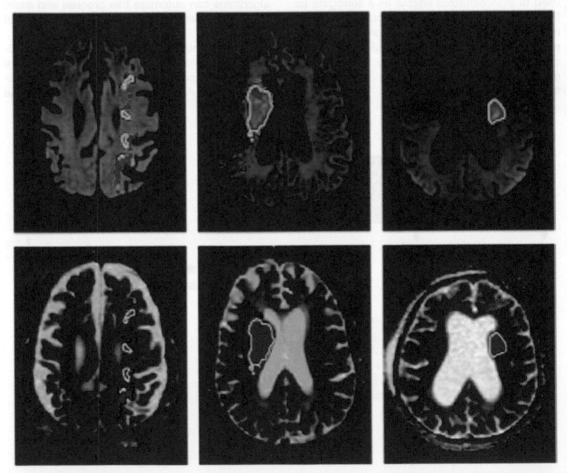

Fig. 5. Qualitative results of infarct segmentation on 3 example cases taken from the independent test set. These cases were picked to illustrate the minimum (*left*), average (*middle*), and maximum Dice similarity coefficient, Hausdorff distance, and volumetric similarity performance of the CNN. The top row includes DWI slices, and the bottom row shows ADC slices. The area in pink is the gold standard for segmentation, the green contours depict the result of automatic segmentation using the proposed U-net architecture.

Therefore, direct implementation of the algorithm without clinical supervision is not advisable at the current level of performance. Further development of the proposed U-Net architecture is necessary before it can be deployed clinically.

Higher acquisition times in MR imaging, especially in the case of DWI imaging, increases its susceptibility to motion-related artifacts such as ghosting, ringing, or blurring as a result of rotation or translation of the head. Most centers deal with motion artifacts by repeating the scans or choosing different sequences to decrease the acquisition times thereby increasing costs, patient burden, and time taken while decreasing quality. Jolink[19] explored the usefulness of deep learning in motion correction for DWI images. This line of research is continuing and is of general applicability in MR imaging.

AUTOMATIC COMPUTED TOMOGRAPHY-BASED STROKE TRIAGE

With multiple randomized controlled trials such as DAWN and DEFUSE 3 demonstrating benefits of endovascular therapy in properly selected patients with acute ischemic stroke, there is a race to build AI tools for rapid triage of these patients. Multiple companies are offering AI platforms that leverage advanced deep learning to process and communicate time-sensitive imaging findings about stroke patients directly to the stroke team. Such platforms hope to harmonize the functioning of multiple, diverse specialties, including neuroradiology, neurology, neurosurgery, and interventional radiology, to synchronize stroke care, decrease time to treatment, and improve access by coordinating care across multiple centers. The model being promoted by these companies is illustrated in Fig. 6.

We briefly describe offerings of 2 leading companies in this space. Both of these companies, Viz.ai and iSchemaView (Menlo Park, CA), produce cloud-based AI platforms for rapid, automatic triage of acute stroke patients.

DETECTION OF LARGE VESSEL OCCLUSIONS

Viz.ai offers an AI-based platform that connects a CT scanner automatically to a cloud-based processing engine. The processing is focused on determining the LVO responsible for acute ischemic stroke, and for generating CTP maps for human and automated analysis. The system automatically segments the neurovascular anatomy to detect sites of suspected LVOs while accounting for vessel bifurcation, retrograde flow through collaterals, and partial occlusions. Based on this processing, stroke specialists are alerted when a positive suspected LVO is detected. If the communication network is appropriately configured, such alerts can go from a spoke hospital to a hub hospital and facilitate integrated stroke care in a spoke-and-hub care model. The stroke team can use a DICOM viewer on a mobile device such as an iPhone to view the site of the LVO. The DICOM viewer is configured for mobile device operation and offers expected facilities such as zooming, scrolling, and window leveling.

Hassan[20] evaluated the impact of Viz.ai system on time between CT angiogram acquisition at a primary stroke center and patient arrival at a comprehensive stroke center. This multicenter, retrospective study compared the transfer time of patients with LVO stroke before and after implementation of Viz.ai. Their analysis showed statistically significant decrease in the transfer time, from 171 minutes to 105 minutes (ie, an average of 66 minutes or 39% time saving; $P = .0163$). This

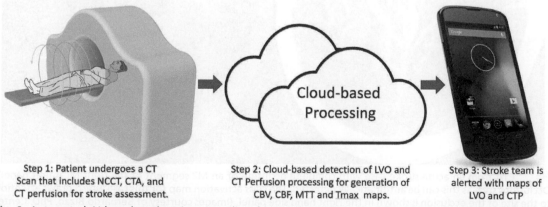

Step 1: Patient undergoes a CT Scan that includes NCCT, CTA, and CT perfusion for stroke assessment.

Step 2: Cloud-based detection of LVO and CT Perfusion processing for generation of CBV, CBF, MTT and Tmax maps.

Step 3: Stroke team is alerted with maps of LVO and CTP

Fig. 6. Automated AI-based stroke triage paradigm being advocated by multiple vendors to decrease the time from detection to endovascular therapy.

study also showed a decrease in the overall length of stay by 2.5 days (P = .0324) and stay in the neuro-intensive care unit by 3.5 days (P = .0039).

Fig. 7 shows a CTA from a stroke case with occlusion of the right middle cerebral artery (MCA). As can be seen, there are very poor collaterals and very few of the M2 and M3 branches of the right MCA are opacified. AI-based software such as Viz LVO, RAPID, and others can automatically flag such cases and alert the stroke team.

RAPID CTA (RAPID 4.9, iSchemaView) is another fully automated AI algorithm approved by the US Food and Drug Administration with high sensitivity for the detection of intracranial anterior circulation LVOs. Amukotuwa and colleagues[21] evaluated the diagnostic accuracy of RAPID CTA with CTAs on 926 patients. The algorithm had a sensitivity of 97% for LVO detection up to the M1 bifurcation, and 95% sensitivity when M2 occlusions were also included. For these scenarios, the specificities were 74% and 70%, respectively. Occlusion site-specific sensitivities were 90% (M1-MCA), 97% (M2-MCA), and 97% (intracranial internal carotid artery) with their corresponding areas under the curve as 0.874, 0.962, and 0.997, respectively.

A slightly lower sensitivity for detection of occlusions in the M2 segments of MCA was attributed to the lower Hounsfield unit decrease in false-negative occlusions. These false negatives were primarily a result of incomplete occlusions that still maintained some antegrade flow of contrast, or they were due to short segment occlusions where collaterals ensured flow distal to the occlusion. A post hoc analysis revealed that the algorithm accurately diagnosed all patients with LVO with poor collateral flow, especially those requiring emergent reperfusion. The high sensitivity of the algorithm enables quick screening for LVOs and rapid mobilization of stroke neurologists and interventional radiologists in case of a positive finding.

CORE AND PENUMBRA ESTIMATION USING COMPUTED TOMOGRAPHY PERFUSION

CTP scanning involves IV injection of iodinated contrast while the brain is being continuously scanned. These time-resolved maps of iodine

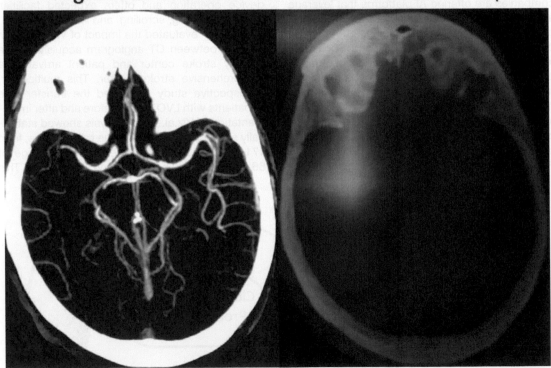

Fig. 7. CTA from an acute stroke case with complete occlusion of an M2 segment of the right MCA (left panel). Occlusions such as this can be automatically detected. The class activation map for this case which draws attention to the site of the occlusion is shown in the right hand side panel. (Images courtesy of Bernardo Bizzo, PhD, Center of Clinical Data Sciences, Massachusetts General Brigham Health Care, Boston, MA; used with author's permission.)

perfusion in and out of brain parenchyma are processed to make maps of cerebral blood flow, cerebral blood volume, mean transit time, and time to peak enhancement. These perfusion maps are used as a surrogate for the delineation of irreversible infarcted tissue, and the tissue that is at risk of infarction if blood flow is not reestablished.

The DEFUSE 3[11] randomized trial evaluated the usefulness of CTP in stroke triage. Its main goal was to assess whether patients with acute ischemic stroke and a CTP measured target mismatch respond favorably to endovascular treatment in a 6- to 16-hour time window after symptom onset compared with standard care alone. The study included patients with symptoms of anterior circulation ischemic stroke, baseline National Institute of Health Stroke Scale (NIHSS) of 6 or greater, last seen to be well 6 to 16 hours previous to the presentation, Modified Rankin Scale of 2 or less before a stroke, and large occlusion of the internal carotid artery or M1-MCA on CTA or MRA. The study used CT scans or MR imaging to define the target mismatch profile as follows: (1) ischemic core volume of less than 70 mL, (2) and mismatch ratio of 1.8 or greater, and a mismatch volume of 15 mL or greater between the penumbra and the core. For patients triaged using CTP, the core was defined as a relative cerebral blood flow of less than 30%, and the penumbra was defined as the time of maximum enhancement of greater than 6 seconds. DEFUSE 3 showed that endovascular thrombectomy in conjunction with standard care for ischemic stroke 6 to 16 hours after onset of symptoms resulted in better 90-day functional outcomes than standard medical therapy alone among patients who had evidence of salvageable tissue.

The DAWN randomized trial[12] compared standard care in acute stroke with endovascular thrombectomy plus standard care in patients within 6 to 24 hours of stroke onset who had a mismatch between clinical deficit and infarct. This study included patients with occlusion of the intracranial internal carotid artery, or the first segment of the MCA, or both seen on CTA, and targeted those with a mismatch between clinical deficit and infarct volume. For inclusion into the thrombectomy arm, the patients had to have a prestroke Modified Rankin Scale score of 0 to 1. The study divided the patients into 3 groups defined as follows:

- Group A: Age 80 years or older, NIHSS of 10 or greater, infarct volume of less than 21 mL;
- Group B: Age less than 80 years; NIHSS of 10 or greater; infarct volume of less than 31 mL;
- Group C: Age less than 80 years; NIHSS of 20 or greater; infarct volume of 31 to 50 mL.

The results of this randomized trial showed that (1) the outcomes in the endovascular therapy arm were better for disability and functional independence, (2) the rate of functional independence was similar to the those treated within 6 hours of symptom onset, and (3) the safety profile of endovascular therapy after 6 to 24 hours was similar to treatment within 6 hours of stroke onset.

Evidence from these 2 trials, and wide availability of CT scanners, has heralded a new era in endovascular therapy for stroke care. Even though Class I, Level A evidence exists for DWI and collateral-based triage for endovascular therapy, CTP is widely used owing to its easy availability: it can be performed on a standard helical CT scanner after the acquisition of noncontrast CT scan and CTA, and a short time is needed to perform it.

Despite its widespread use, CTP has several drawbacks that should be kept in mind. CTP imaging suffers from variability in perfusion maps across vendors, difficulties in standardized assessment, and a high radiation dose for the patient.[22] Other drawbacks include a limited usefulness in situations with poor cardiac output, atrial fibrillation, large proximal occlusion (which generate inaccurate perfusion maps), variability in acquisition methods and interpretation, and above all, lack of proper validation against any gold standard for core and penumbra.[23]

Fig. 8 shows a CTA from a stroke case with occlusion of the left MCA. As can be seen, there are very poor collaterals and very few of the M2 and M3 branches of the left MCA are opacified. (The apparent cut off of the P1 segment of the right PCA, with the distal portions well opacified, is an artifact of MIP slice selection.) AI-based software such as Viz LVO, RAPID, and others can automatically flag such cases and alert the stroke team.

Multiple software packages from CT scanner manufacturers and independent companies are available for generating CTP maps. Majority of them are automated or require minimal human supervision. Fig. 9 shows the CTP maps for the stroke patient whose CTA was presented in Fig. 8.

CHALLENGES AND FUTURE DIRECTIONS

Stroke imaging provides a fertile ground for AI research. Conversely, AI tools provide a solution to some of most vexing problems in stroke care, which include geographic mismatch between patients and comprehensive stroke centers, a stringent timeline that must be adhered to in stroke care, and the need for cloud computing coupled

NCCT   CTA (from CTP run)

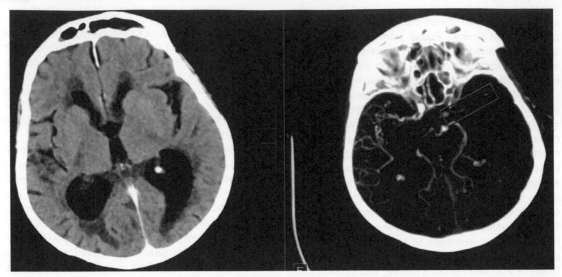

Fig. 8. CTA from an acute stroke case with complete occlusion of the M1 segment of the left MCA. There are very poor collaterals in this territory.

with efficient communication. So it is expected that there will be continued symbiotic interplay between AI tools and stroke care.

There are multiple challenges, however, that must be addressed for this relationship to grow and produce even more significant contributions. First and foremost is the challenge of siloed health care data. AI algorithms are data hungry and the veracity of their output crucially depends on the training set used to train them. If the training set consists of data that embody the heterogeneity and unpredictability of routine clinical situations, the AI algorithm will behave appropriately. However, in the absence of such training data, it can fail in inexplicable ways.

Unfortunately, most deep learning algorithms that are deployed have been trained and validated with limited data when one compares the size of

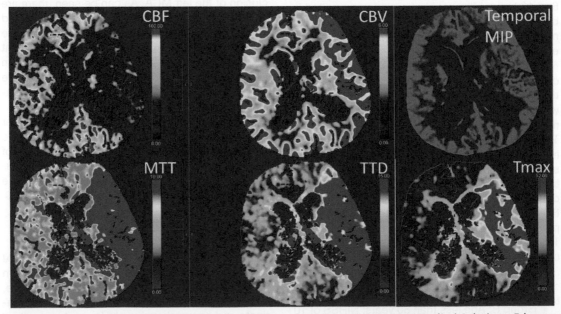

Fig. 9. CTP maps for the case shown in **Fig. 8**, processed using Singo.via (Siemens Medical Solutions, Erlangen, Germany). CBF, cerebral blood flow; CBV, cerebral blood volume; MTT, mean transit time; T_{max}, time of maximum enhancement; TTD, time to drain; Temporal MIP, temporal maximum intensity projection.

medical datasets with those in social networking, Internet applications, automated driving, and other endeavors where the Health Insurance Portability and Accountability Act and privacy concerns are not as stringent as in health care. The quality and size of the datasets influence the results and can lead to poor generalizability of the trained networks. From this point of view, creation of large, multinational and multi-institutional datasets, such as the Ischemic Stroke Lesion Segmentation Challenge[24] and the RSNA Brain Hemorrhage CT dataset,[25] are a welcome step in the right direction. Such public efforts provide large and diverse datasets for the training, testing, and validation of deep learning algorithms for greater generalizability. Further efforts should focus on consolidating such datasets to include scans of complex and varied pathologies, including scans from both ambulatory and emergent settings. They should also include heterogeneous ethnicities, races, scanner types, institutions, and countries.

A lack of standards for demonstrating generalizability, clinical validity, and reporting are some other challenges to AI in stroke imaging and in neuroradiology as a whole. Area under the curve, the Dice similarity coefficient, Hausdorff distance, sensitivity, and specificity are some of the commonly used metrics for assessing and reporting deep learning algorithms. These metrics, however, tend to be highly dependent on the test set used for vetting the algorithm. The absence of standardized reporting parameters makes the interpretation and comparison of various AI algorithms a challenge.

In addition to these problems with validation and reporting the veracity of an AI algorithm, there is a fundamental issue in training itself. A trained CNN carries the biases of the training set. For example, if a certain pathology is overrepresented as compared with another, the network will have a tendency to bias the answer toward the more frequent pathology. There is no clear mechanism or theory that guides how one can create a balanced dataset for training.

Finally, models and codes developed by AI researchers and companies are not available openly for validation. This factor leads to limited reproducibility of the findings and limited ability to validate using external data. The disconnect between AI scientists and physicians, which may contribute to inadequate clinical validation of various models, may also act as a barrier to the effective integration of AI in clinical practice. A growing collaboration between AI researchers, computer scientists, and physicians is a hopeful sign in bridging these gaps and allowing for the effective integration of AI in clinical practice.

In summary, although these shortcomings are significant, they are not insurmountable. Efforts should be made to overcome them, considering the huge potential benefits of AI in stroke imaging and medicine in general.

DISCLOSURE

The authors have nothing to disclose.

REFERENCES

1. Parsons M, Spratt N, Bivard A, et al. A randomized trial of tenecteplase versus alteplase for acute ischemic stroke. N Engl J Med 2012;366(12): 1099–107. https://doi.org/10.1056/NEJMoa1109842.
2. Hacke W, Kaste M, Bluhmki E, et al. Thrombolysis with Alteplase 3 to 4.5 hours after acute ischemic stroke. N Engl J Med 2008;359(13):1317–29. https://doi.org/10.1056/NEJMoa0804656.
3. Campbell BCV, Mitchell PJ, Churilov L, et al. Tenecteplase versus Alteplase before thrombectomy for ischemic stroke. N Engl J Med 2018;378(17): 1573–82. https://doi.org/10.1056/NEJMoa1716405.
4. Logallo N, Novotny V, Assmus J, et al. Tenecteplase versus alteplase for management of acute ischaemic stroke (NOR-TEST): a phase 3, randomised, open-label, blinded endpoint trial. Lancet Neurol 2017;16(10):781–8. https://doi.org/10.1016/S1474-4422(17)30253-3.
5. von Kummer R, Mori E, Truelsen T, et al. Desmoteplase 3 to 9 hours after major artery occlusion stroke: the DIAS-4 trial (efficacy and safety study of desmoteplase to treat acute ischemic stroke). Stroke 2016;47(12):2880–7. https://doi.org/10.1161/STROKEAHA.116.013715.
6. Berkhemer OA, Fransen PSS, Beumer D, et al. A randomized trial of intraarterial treatment for acute ischemic stroke. N Engl J Med 2015;372(1):11–20. https://doi.org/10.1056/NEJMoa1411587.
7. Jovin TG, Chamorro A, Cobo E, et al. Thrombectomy within 8 hours after symptom onset in ischemic stroke. N Engl J Med 2015;372(24):2296–306. https://doi.org/10.1056/NEJMoa1503780.
8. Goyal M, Demchuk AM, Menon BK, et al. Randomized assessment of rapid endovascular treatment of ischemic stroke. N Engl J Med 2015;372(11): 1019–30. https://doi.org/10.1056/NEJMoa1414905.
9. Campbell BCV, Mitchell PJ, Kleinig TJ, et al. Endovascular therapy for ischemic stroke with perfusion-imaging selection. N Engl J Med 2015; 372(11):1009–18. https://doi.org/10.1056/NEJMoa1414792.
10. Saver JL, Goyal M, Bonafe A, et al. Stent-retriever thrombectomy after intravenous t-PA vs. t-PA alone

in stroke. N Engl J Med 2015;372(24):2285–95. https://doi.org/10.1056/NEJMoa1415061.

11. Albers GW, Marks MP, Kemp S, et al. Thrombectomy for stroke at 6 to 16 hours with selection by perfusion imaging. N Engl J Med 2018;378(8):708–18. https://doi.org/10.1056/NEJMoa1713973.

12. Nogueira RG, Jadhav AP, Haussen DC, et al. Thrombectomy 6 to 24 hours after stroke with a mismatch between deficit and infarct. N Engl J Med 2018; 378(1):11–21.   https://doi.org/10.1056/NEJMoa1706442.

13. Leslie-Mazwi TM, Lev MH. Towards artificial intelligence for clinical stroke care. Nat Rev Neurol 2020;16(1):5–6.   https://doi.org/10.1038/s41582-019-0287-9.

14. Wada R, Aviv RI, Fox AJ, et al. CT angiography "spot sign" predicts hematoma expansion in acute intracerebral hemorrhage. Stroke 2007;38(4):1257–62. https://doi.org/10.1161/01.STR.0000259633.59404.f3.

15. Lipman K. Deep learning-based prediction of intracerebral hemorrhage expansion with Dual-Energy Computed Tomography. Oral Presentation presented at the: ASNR 2020, 58th Annual Meeting; June 30, 2020; Las Vegas, NV.

16. Metselaar R, Bergmans R, Jolink F, et al. Synthetic MR DWI images based on CT imaging in acute ischemic stroke patients. Enschede (the Netherlands): University of Twente; 2019.

17. Merino JG, Warach S. Imaging of acute stroke. Nat Rev Neurol 2010;6(10):560–71. https://doi.org/10.1038/nrneurol.2010.129.

18. Hamelink I, Gupta R. Multimodal U-Net for ischemic stroke lesion segmentation in DWI and ADC.

Enschede (the Netherlands): University of Twente; 2019.

19. Jolink FC. Deep learning based reduction of motion artifacts in DWI 2020.

20. Hassan AE, Ringheanu VM, Rabah R, et al. Abstract TMP62: early experience utilizing artificial intelligence shows significant reduction in transfer times and length of stay in a hub and spoke model. Stroke 2020;51(Suppl_1):ATMP62. https://doi.org/10.1161/str.51.suppl_1.TMP62.

21. Amukotuwa SA, Straka M, Dehkharghani S, et al. Fast automatic detection of large vessel occlusions on CT angiography. Stroke 2019;50(12):3431–8. https://doi.org/10.1161/STROKEAHA.119.027076.

22. Borst J, Berkhemer OA, Roos YBWEM, et al. Value of computed tomographic perfusion-based patient selection for intra-arterial acute ischemic stroke treatment. Stroke 2015;46(12):3375–82. https://doi.org/10.1161/STROKEAHA.115.010564.

23. González RG, Copen WA, Schaefer PW, et al. The Massachusetts General Hospital acute stroke imaging algorithm: an experience and evidence based approach. J Neurointerventional Surg 2013;5(Suppl 1):i7–12. https://doi.org/10.1136/neurintsurg-2013-010715.

24. Yao AD, Cheng DL, Pan I, et al. Deep learning in neuroradiology: a systematic review of current algorithms and approaches for the new wave of imaging technology. Radiol Artif Intell 2020;2(2):e190026. https://doi.org/10.1148/ryai.2020190026.

25. Flanders AE, Prevedello LM, Shih G, et al. Construction of a machine learning dataset through collaboration: the RSNA 2019 brain CT hemorrhage challenge. Radiol Artif Intell 2020;2(3):e190211. https://doi.org/10.1148/ryai.2020190211.

Artificial Intelligence and Stroke Imaging
A West Coast Perspective

Guangming Zhu, MD, PhD, Bin Jiang, MD, PhD, Hui Chen, MD, PhD,
Elizabeth Tong, MD, PhD, Yuan Xie, PhD, Tobias D. Faizy, MD, PhD,
Jeremy J. Heit, MD, PhD, Greg Zaharchuk, MD, PhD,
Max Wintermark, MD, MAS*

KEYWORDS

• Artificial intelligence • Machine learning • Deep learning • Stroke imaging

KEY POINTS

- There is an important need to rapidly and precisely interpret neuroimaging data in stroke, with many potential artificial intelligence (AI) applications.
- AI has the potential to help neuroradiologists.
- More standardized imaging data sets and more extensive AI studies are needed to establish and validate the role of AI in stroke imaging.

INTRODUCTION

Artificial intelligence (AI) is a branch of computer science that has seen dramatic developments in the past couple years, and these AI advancements have significant implications for medical imaging. AI increasingly is able to perform accurate lesion classification, detection, and segmentation in a variety of organs and tissue types. AI also has been used for imaging-guided decision making and outcome prediction. There are many excellent reviews of AI in radiology, covering topics ranging from medical imaging[1–7] and neuroradiology[8–12] to stroke imaging,[13–16] and from imaging techniques[8] to imaging-based outcome prediction.[9,17] This article focuses on the application of AI to stroke imaging.

Stroke is the leading cause of disability and the fifth leading cause of death in the United States. There are vast amounts of stroke imaging data and a large number of multidisciplinary approaches used in making clinical decisions. AI techniques are well-suited for dealing with this large amount of data, and AI applications for stroke imaging are a topic of intense research. AI algorithms may detect and quantify intracranial hemorrhage (ICH), microbleeds, chronic ischemic white matter disease, and acute ischemic stroke (AIS), which includes the presence of cerebral infarction and large vessel occlusions.[18,19] The time interval between the onset of AIS and its diagnosis/treatment often is vital for a favorable clinical outcome. Therefore, AI solutions for stroke imaging need to be very time efficient.

According to a review by Lee and colleagues,[16] until 2017, only a limited number of publications existed dealing with machine learning (ML) applied to stroke imaging. Sakai and Yamada[10] reviewed ML studies applied to major brain diseases from 2014 to 2018. They found only 7 stroke imaging studies based on ML, with stroke ranking tenth in terms of topic of AI studies, after Alzheimer disease, mild cognitive impairment, brain tumor, schizophrenia, and others. None of the 7 studies was based on large data sets. There are many companies developing AI-based imaging applications, utilizing ML and deep learning (DL) models for the diagnosis and management of various

Department of Neuroradiology, Stanford University, 300 Pasteur Drive, Stanford, CA 94305, USA
* Corresponding author.
E-mail address: max.wintermark@gmail.com
Twitter: @mwNRAD (M.W.)

Neuroimag Clin N Am 30 (2020) 479–492
https://doi.org/10.1016/j.nic.2020.07.001

diseases, but only a few of them are focusing on stroke imaging.

The authors performed a PubMed search covering the past 5 years and found 766 publications addressing AI for neuroimaging, 35 publications addressing AI for stroke, and only 66 publications reporting of AI and stroke imaging. The time for publication inclusion was from September 26, 2014, to September 25, 2019. Keywords used included ("Artificial Intelligence" OR "Deep Learning (DL)" OR "Machine Learning" OR "Neuron Network" OR "Random Forest (RF)" OR "Support Vector Machine (SVM)" OR "Decision Tree" OR "Naïve Bayes") AND ("Stroke" OR "Stroke imaging" OR "Stroke image" OR "Brain Imaging" OR "Neuroimaging" OR Neuroradiology"). The number of studies found showed a significant increase over the course of the 5 years (Fig. 1). The authors also reviewed the type of AI algorithms used in these studies. A majority of them were based on DL algorithms, such as neural networks, especially since 2019 (Fig. 2). Selected publications dealing with AI-based stroke imaging are listed in Table 1.

ARTIFICIAL INTELLIGENCE APPLICATIONS FOR THE ACQUISITION AND POSTPROCESSING OF STROKE IMAGING DATA

AI has been applied to a wide range of tasks related to stroke imaging. Many AI applications have focused on the downstream side of imaging evaluation, which includes lesion detection, segmentation, treatment decision support, and outcome prediction. Many innovative AI applications, however, also have tackled upstream applications, such as modulation of imaging techniques used. AI can be used to reduce the gadolinium dose in contrast-enhanced brain magnetic resonance imaging (MRI) or the radiation dose in computed tomography (CT) and PET, without significant reductions in image quality.[33,68,69] AI also can be used for undersampled data sets to generate quality images. For instance, Gibbons and colleagues[22] proposed a convolutional neural network (CNN) model to generate diffusion spectrum imaging (DSI). This model provided a 10-fold reduction scan time and the poststroke outcome prediction metrics were comparable to conventional imaging.

A recent study established a new parametric model using a deep CNN for dynamic contrast-enhanced (DCE) MRI. Tracer kinetic models, such as the Patlak model and extended Tofts model,[70] traditionally have been used to extract pharmacokinetic parameters from DCE MRI, in order to characterize vascular permeability and tissue perfusion. Both have the limitation of noisy postprocessing with large variance. Ulas and colleagues[20] utilized a deep CNN and applied it to DCE MRI obtained in mild ischemic stroke patients to learn the mapping between the image-time series and the corresponding pharmacokinetic parameters extracted from conventional processing. The CNN method enabled a faster and more robust parameter inference.[20]

Another study by Kim and colleagues[21] demonstrated image quality improvement for pseudo-continuous ASL. They used data with 2 signal averages to predict images acquired with 6 signal averages, an approximately 3-fold speed-up in imaging time. Using this CNN DL algorithm, it also was possible to reconstruct Hadamard-encoded ASL imaging from a subset of the reconstructed postlabel delay images.

Other AI applications for image acquisition include image artifact reduction, improving image resolution, and shortening image acquisition duration. Although most of these applications were not applied specifically to stroke imaging, they are adaptable to this clinical problem.[8]

DIAGNOSIS APPROACH: AUTOMATIC LESION IDENTIFICATION AND/OR SEGMENTATION

Neuroimaging is a cornerstone of the work-up of AIS patients. Interpretation of neuroimaging in stroke patients is challenging, however, especially in the hyperacute phase when imaging findings of stroke are subtle. AI has the potential to help with some of these diagnostic challenges.

Computer-Aided Diagnosis and Computer-Aided Simple Triage

In the 1980s, a concept named computer-aided diagnosis (CAD) was introduced to provide radiologists with a second opinion regarding their image interpretation.[71] With the development of AI over the past few years, CAD was transitioned to computer-aided simple triage (CAST). CAST performs a fully automated analysis of medical images and then provides an initial classification.[72] It is meant to attract a physician's attention to critical and time-sensitive findings, such as an AIS. AI-based CAD or CAST may optimize the stroke imaging workflow, facilitate earlier diagnosis, and prompt communication of critical findings. Titano and colleagues[28] combined CNN with natural language processing (NLP) to identify a broad range of acute neurologic illnesses, including stroke, ICH, and hydrocephalus. The investigators stated that "with a total processing and interpretation time of 1.2 seconds, such a triage system can alert physicians to a critical finding that may otherwise

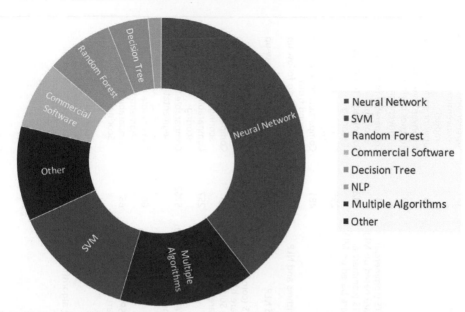

Fig. 1. Five-year trends of AI-based stroke imaging, stroke, and neuroimaging studies.

remain in a queue for minutes to hours." Commercial platforms are available that send an alert within 6 minutes if a patient is suspected of having a large vessel occlusion stroke.[18]

Chilamkurthy and colleagues[27] collected 313,318 noncontrast head CT (NCCT) scans and developed DL algorithms to detect critical findings on these NCCT scans, including ICH, fracture, midline shift, and mass effect. The best area under the curve (AUC) was for the detection of ICH, which was at approximately 0.94. For the detection of mass effect on the brain, the AUC was above 0.85. Prevedello and colleagues[26] proposed a CNN model to detect critical findings on NCCT. For hemorrhage, mass effect, and hydrocephalus, the detection was highly accurate with AUC of 0.91, whereas the detection of suspected acute infarct was relatively less accurate, although still reasonable, with an AUC of 0.81.[26]

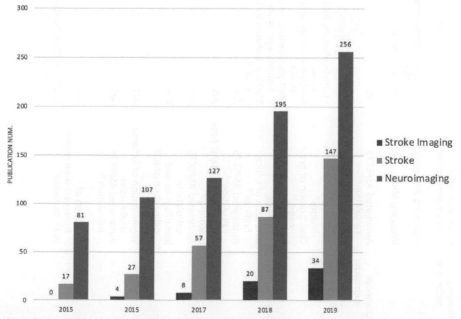

Fig. 2. AI algorithms used in stroke imaging studies. NUM, number.

Table 1
Selected artificial intelligence studies on stroke imaging within past 5 years

Purpose	Detail	Setting	Imaging Modality	Imaging Parameters	Artificial Intelligence Classifier	Number of Subjects	Performance
Imaging techniques	Pharmacokinetic parameters estimate[20]	Chronic ischemic stroke	MRI	DCE	CNN	15	Superior performance over conventional fitting model
	Improving ASL quality[21]	Multiple diseases, including stroke	MRI	ASL-CBF	CNN	14	Superior performance over conventional methods
	Reducing MRI scan time[22]	Subacute stroke	MRI	DSI	CNN	29	Superior performance over conventional methods
Diagnosis approach	Automated ASPECTS calculation[23]	AIS	CT	NCCT	e-ASPECTS (commercial software based on ML)	34	Comparable to manual scoring
	Automated ASPECTS calculation[24]	AIS	CT	NCCT	e-ASPECTS (commercial software based on ML)	132	Comparable to manual scoring
	Classification of brain images[25]	Multiple diseases, including stroke	CT	NCCT	CNN	285	Comparable to ground truth
	Classification of brain images[26]	Multiple diseases, including stroke	CT	NCCT	CNN	481	Comparable to follow-up ground truth
	Detection of critical findings[27]	Multiple diseases, including hemorrhagic stroke	CT	NCCT	DL algorithms and NLP	313,318	Comparable to follow-up ground truth
	Detection of critical findings[28]	Multiple diseases, including stroke	CT	NCCT	CNN and NLP	37,236	Comparable to follow-up ground truth
	Automated ASPECTS calculation[29]	AIS	CT	NCCT	e-APECTS (commercial software based on ML)	119	Comparable to manual scoring
	Automated collateral flow scoring[30]	AIS	CT	CTA	e-Stroke Suite (commercial software based on ML)	98	Comparable to manual scoring
	Automated ASPECTS calculation[31]	AIS	CT	NCCT	RF	257	Comparable to manual scoring
	Identification and delineation of ICH lesion[32]	ICH	CT	NCCT	CNN + feedforward neural network	5702	Comparable to manual segmentation
	Segmentation of ischemic stroke lesion[33]	AIS	CT	CTA-SIs	CNN	60	Comparable to manual segmentation
	Automated ASPECTS dalculation[34]	AIS	CT and MRI	NCCT, DWI	Rapid ASPECTS (commercial software based on ML)	65	Comparable to manual Scoring
	Detection of hyperperfusion region[35]	AIS	MRI	ASL-CBF	CNN	361 scans	Comparable to manual segmentation
	ISLES challenge[36]	Subacute ischemic stroke and AIS	MRI	T1, T1+C, T2, DWI, PWI (CBV, CBF, Tmax, TTP), FLAIR	Multiple algorithms: RF, CNN	114	Comparable to manual segmentation
	Brain lesion segmentation[37]	Multiple diseases, including stroke	MRI	T1, T1+C, FLAIR, DWI	CNN	384	Comparable to manual segmentation

Application	Condition	Modality	Sequence	Algorithm	n	Result
Segmentation of infarct lesion[38]	Subacute ischemic stroke	MR	DWI, T1, T2, FLAIR	Autoencoder CNN and SVM	28	Comparable to manual segmentation
Brain lesion segmentation[39]	Stroke and tumor	MRI	T1+C, T2, DWI, PWI (CBV, CBF, Tmax, TTP)	RF and RBM (restricted Boltzmann machine)	115	Comparable to manual segmentation
Segmentation of infarct lesion[40]	AIS	MRI	ADC, DWI	Decision tree	108	Comparable to manual segmentation
Segmentation of infarct lesion[41]	Chronic ischemic stroke	MRI	T1, T2, FLAIR	SVM and RF	200	Comparable to manual classification
Determination of stroke onset time[42]	AIS	MR	DWI, ADC, PWI (CBV, CBF, MTT, TTP, Tmax), FLAIR,	Autoencoder CNN and multiple ML algorithms	131	Superior performance over conventional DWI-FLAIR mismatch
Identify brain MRI report[43]	Multiple diseases, including stroke	MRI	MRI report	Multiple ML algorithms	3204	Comparable to final diagnosis
Rapid clot analysis[44]	AIS	MRI	GRE	Multiple ML algorithms	67	Comparable to ground truth
Automated microbleed detection[45]	Multiple diseases, including stroke	MR	SWI	CNN	154	Comparable to manual detection
WMH burden quantification[46]	AIS	MRI	FLAIR	Autoencoder CNN	144	Comparable to manual segmentation
Vessel segmentation[47]	Steno-occlusive cerebrovascular disease	MR	TOF	CNN with U-Net	82	Comparable to manual segmentation
Segmentation of hematoma[48]	ICH	MR	GRE, FLAIR	Self-built algorithm vs CNN	50	Comparable results with CNN DL method.
Lesion segmentation to phenotype AIS[49]	AIS	MR	ADC, DWI	CNN	3680	Comparable to manual detection
Segmentation of infarct lesion[50]	AIS	MR	ADC, DWI	CNN with U-Net	430	Comparable to manual classification and commercial software based on ML (Rapid)
Brain lesion segmentation[51]	Multiple diseases, including stroke	MRI	FLAIR	CNN with U-Net	38	Comparable to manual segmentation
Carotid wall plaque morphology to predict stroke risk[52]	Diabetic patients with stroke risk	U/S		SVM	407 scans	Comparable to manual segmentation
Carotid intima-media thickness measurement[53]	Diabetic patients with stroke risk	U/S		CNN	396 scans	Comparable to manual segmentation
Carotid lumen detection[54]	Diabetic patients with stroke risk	U/S		CNN	407 scans	Superior performance over conventional methods
Carotid plaque segmentation[55]	Carotid stenosis >60%	U/S		CNN with U-Net and dynamic CNN	144	Comparable to manual segmentation

(continued on next page)

Table 1
(continued)

Purpose	Detail	Setting	Imaging Modality	Imaging Parameters	Artificial Intelligence Classifier	Number of Subjects	Performance
Prognosis approach	Predict SICH after thrombolysis[56]	AIS	CT	NCCT	SVM	116	Comparable to ground truth
	Predict the infarct volume growth[57]	AIS	CT	CTP (CBV, TTD)	CNN with U-Net	29	Comparable to manual segmentation
	Predict ischemic core[58]	AIS	CT	CTP (CBV, CBF, Tmax, TTP)	ANN	128	Comparable to follow-up ground truth
	Make treatment decision[59]	AIS	CT	CTP (CBV, CBF, MTT, Tmax)	RF	80	Comparable to follow-up ground truth
	Predict the thrombolysis functional outcomes[60]	AIS	CT	NCCT	CNN and ANN	204	Comparable to follow-up ground truth
	Predict the final infarct volume[61]	AIS	MRI	Raw PWI	SVM	4	Comparable to follow-up ground truth
	Predict the final infarct volume[62]	AIS	MRI	DWI, FLAIR, PWI (CBV, TTP, MTT, Tmax)	XGB	195	Comparable to follow-up ground truth
	Predict the final infarct volume[63]	AIS	MRI	Raw PWI	CNN	48	Comparable to follow-up ground truth
	Predict the lesion outcome[64]	AIS	MRI	ADC, PWI (CBV, CBF, MTT, TTP, Tmax)	CNN with U-Net	75	Comparable to follow-up ground truth
	Predict the clinical outcome[65]	AIS	MRI	DTI	SVM	87	Comparable to follow-up ground truth
	Predict cognitive performance[66]	AIS	MRI	T1, T2, FLAIR	CNN and multiple ML algorithm	153	Comparable to follow-up ground truth
	Ischemic stroke lesion outcome prediction challenge 2016[67]	AIS	MRI	ADC, PWI (CBV, CBF, MTT, Tmax, TTP), and raw PWI	CNN	64	Comparable to follow-up ground truth
	Ischemic stroke lesion outcome prediction challenge 2017[67]	AIS	MRI	ADC, PWI (CBV, CBF, MTT, Tmax, TTP), and raw PWI	CNN	75	Comparable to follow-up ground truth

Abbreviations: ASL, arterial spin labeling; CBF, cerebral blood flow; CBV, cerebral blood volume; MTT, mean transit time; PWI, perfusion weighted imaging; RBM, restricted boltzmann machine; SICH, symptomatic intracerebral hemorrhage; T1, T1 weighted imaging; T1+C, T1 weighted imaging with contrast; T2, T2 weighted imaging; Tmax, time to maximum; TTD, time to drain; TTP, time to peak; U/S, ultrasound.

The time from stroke onset is another crucial factor for making stroke treatment decisions. Stroke patients with unknown or unwitnessed onset often are excluded from early aggressive therapy, such as thrombolysis and thrombectomy. Many tissue clock methods, for example, the diffusion-weighted imaging (DWI)-fluid-attenuated inversion recovery (FLAIR) mismatch,[73] are used to estimate the time from stroke onset, but these approaches suffer from relatively poor performances.[74] Ho and colleagues[42] proposed an autoencoder CNN DL model to extract hidden features from routine and perfusion MRI, then used 5 ML models to classify the time since stroke onset less than 4.5 hours. The cross-validation results showed an AUC of 0.765, outperforming the concurrent DWI-FLAIR mismatch method.[42]

Although CAD and CAST developers focus on modalities used in the emergency diagnostic setting, many studies also use CAD for chronic and nonemergent conditions. Gao and colleagues[25] utilized a CNN DL architecture to classify NCCT. They clustered 3 categories of NCCT, including Alzheimer disease, lesion (tumor, stroke, and so forth), and normal aging. The classification accuracy rates for Alzheimer disease and normal aging were 85.2% and 95.3%, respectively, much better than for lesion detection (80%).[25]

Lesion Detection and Characterization

Lesion detection in stroke imaging increasingly is focused not only on the detection of cerebral ischemia but also in guiding stroke treatment. For example, patients with AIS due to a large vessel occlusion potentially are candidates for endovascular thrombectomy. Therefore, AI approaches to identify the presence of a large vessel occlusion through the automated detection of the hyperdense artery dense/dot sign on NCCT, which represents the arterial clot causing the stroke, are important. Takahashi and colleagues[75] implemented regions of interest around the sylvian fissure regions, identifying middle cerebral artery (MCA) dots, and then classified images using an SVM with 4 features. The algorithm performed with a sensitivity of 97.5% (39/40) and a false-positive rate of 50% (54/109).[75]

MCA dots on NCCT show up as blooming artifacts on MRI. Chung and colleagues[44] developed an ML-based automated and rapid clot analysis system to detect clots within the MCA, which also was able to predict the source of the clots to be atrial fibrillation by evaluating the clots' imaging characteristics.

The Alberta Stroke Program Early CT Score (ASPECTS) is an established 10-point quantitative topographic CT scan score, which has been used widely to assess the extent of early ischemic changes on brain imaging for acute stroke treatment decision. ASPECTS may suffer, however, from a significant interobserver variability. e-ASPECTS is a standardized, fully automated ASPECTS scoring tool for NCCT, based on an ML algorithm. This software system has been applied in multiple studies,[23,24,29] all suggesting noninferiority of the computer tool to experienced neuroradiologists in applying the ASPECTS to NCCTs of AIS patients.

The robustness of collaterals in the context of ischemic stroke due to large vessel occlusion is an important factor for endovascular thrombectomy treatment candidacy. Similar to other scoring systems, CT angiography (CTA) collateral scoring often is inconsistent between raters. The CTA module uses a combination of classical image processing techniques and ML classifiers to categorize the degree of collateral flow in real time and in a fully automated fashion. Grunwald and colleagues[30] performed a study to evaluate this module's performance and the results demonstrated a high degree of agreement between the fully automated and objective e-CTA score and a consensus expert CTA–collateral scoring approach.[30,76]

There are many other medical imaging systems based on ML. One significant limitation of ML based systems is their dependence on feature extraction techniques. Extracting features is a time-consuming process, and some conditions may not be associated with recognizable features to the human eye.[2] The advantage of DL systems is that they can generate their own features and are independent from feature extraction techniques. Also, their greater depth allows them to learn complex functions and composite relationships between data components. For all these reasons, there is a trend to more and more shift the focus of AI systems to DL.

Lesion Segmentation

Segmentation is a common task in medical image analysis, which is different from detecting lesions. As lesion detection focuses on marking potential abnormalities, segmentation focuses on delineating the abnormalities. It provides valuable information for the analysis of brain damage and may play a role for treatment selection, monitoring disease progression, and outcome prediction. Although a variety of ML algorithms have been used[39–41] for lesion segmentation, many have failed to demonstrate superiority over human manual segmentation.[77–79] In terms of stroke, this is attributed to the variable appearance of the ischemic lesions on NCCT and MRIs, also depending on time of stroke onset, the affected vascular territory, and collateral flow status. In addition, different noise signals, such as leukoaraiosis, T2 shine-through effect, and distinct tissue effects also can impede a successful lesion segmentation. In general, DL algorithms based on CNN are more promising versus SVM, RF, and others, so that they have been more widely applied over the recent years.

Generally, there are 2 kinds of segmentation strategies. The first uses a 2-step process: (1) to make a rough estimate, usually with a DL framework, and (2) to tune for a finer segmentation with either DL framework or conventional ML methods. The second approach is either to FCN for semantic segmentation or to divide the images into very small patches as labels, which are reassembled to give the segmentation mask of the given images.

Lesion segmentation on NCCT for AIS is a challenging task, but the segmentation of ICH is easier given the greater density discrepancy between hemorrhage and the normal brain. Some algorithms use ML-based approaches, for instance RF.[80] Because DL algorithms, that is, CNN, enable self-learning of nonlinear image filters and self-extraction of relevant features, they are more suitable for segmentation. Cho and colleagues[32] constructed a cascade DL model with CNN and FCN. CNN was used to identify bleeding, and FCN was used to classify 5 different subtypes of ICH and delineate these lesions. In determining the presence of cerebral hemorrhage, the algorithm showed a robust 97.91% sensitivity and 98.76% specificity. For delineation of ICH, the overall segmentation performance was 80.19% in precision and 82.15% in recall.

NCCT has a relatively low sensitivity for acute brain ischemia in the first 12 hours of stroke. Other CT modalities, including CT perfusion (CTP) and CTA, are used to increase sensitivity to acute brain ischemia and select potential candidates who are suitable for early aggressive therapy. The hypoattenuation on CTA source images (CTA-SIs) can provide an estimate of the cerebral blood volume reduction and of the ischemic core. Öman and colleagues[33] applied 3-dimensional (3-D)–CNN (CNN) to detect ischemic stroke on CTA-SIs and then segment the lesion. The performance of volumetric diagnosis on CTA-SIs achieved an AUC of 0.93 with Dice similarity coefficient of 0.61.[33]

MRI, especially DWI, is most suitable for early detection of ischemic stroke lesions. Therefore, most automated segmentation algorithms of AIS are applying DWI. Kim and colleagues[50] adopted an encoder-decoder CNN (U-net) to train segmentation models on DWI and apparent diffusion coefficient (ADC) data. When compared with expert's manual segmentation, the testing performance of U-net showed a high correlation with the expert measurements.[50] Wu and colleagues[49] utilized DeepMedic framework (3-D–CNN) to segment acute ischemic lesions on heterogeneous multicenter clinical DWI MRI data sets. The subset analysis comparing automated and manual lesion volumes in 383 patients found an excellent correlation ($P = 0.92$; $P<.0001$)[49] between both approaches.

White matter hyperintensity (WMH) burden is linked to vascular risk factor and predisposes patients to vascular dementia. Schirmer and colleagues[46] obtained WMH volumes by building on an automatic WMH segmentation algorithm based on CNN. It can match expert knowledge of the spatial distribution of the WMH burden and demonstrate the increase of WMH burden with age (0.950 cm^3/y). Other examples of MRI studies include vessel segmentation on time of flight (TOF),[47] hematoma segmentation on gradient echo (GRE),[48] and multiple brain lesion segmentation on FLAIR.[51]

In summary, manual segmentation is cumbersome and inconsistent across raters. The implementation of image-classifier AI algorithms, especially CNN DL algorithms, can be used to classify each individual voxel in the image. With the powerful computing capacity of modern graphics processing units, AI allows such a task to be achieved automatically and efficiently.

Artificial Intelligence and Other Imaging Tools

Besides MRI and CT, AI also can be applied to other stroke imaging modalities, such as ultrasound. Gray-scale morphology of the ultrasound carotid wall can be used for the classification of high-risk plaques versus low-risk plaques or for symptomatic plaques versus asymptomatic plaques. It is challenging, however, to characterize a plaque visually, given the wide variation in ultrasound technique and the operator dependency of the images. Biswas and colleagues published multiple studies using AI techniques for automatic carotid ultrasound analysis.[53] The investigators used ML and DL algorithms separately to automatically segment carotid wall and detect plaques. Both ML and DL algorithms suggested good results with AUC greater than 0.90. The investigators, however, did not compare the performance between ML and DL algorithms.[52–54]

PROGNOSIS APPROACH: PREDICTION OF TREATMENT COMPLICATIONS AND CLINICAL OUTCOMES
Prediction of Tissue Fate

Acute stroke results in high morbidity and mortality. It is crucial to assess possible outcome and make an appropriate treatment decision in a timely fashion, especially for AIS with large vessel occlusion. This decision often is influenced by a combination of data derived from randomized trials and the treating physician's personal experience. More objective approaches, like using imaging guidance to confirm the eligibility of AIS patients for thrombolytic therapy or endovascular mechanical thrombectomy, have started to become part of the standard of care. There is a great need for advanced data analysis techniques that identify the target mismatch between the ischemic core and the salvageable penumbra and predict tissue outcome in a reproducible and accurate way.

Kasasbeh and colleagues[58] utilized artificial neural networks (ANNs) based on CTP and/or clinical data to predict the ischemic core in AIS patients, using DWI as the ground truth. The AUC was 0.85 on CTP data only and 0.87 on CTP with clinical data. The maximal Dice coefficient was 0.48.[58] Lucas and colleagues[57] suggested that even highly complex AI algorithms are not fully capable of directly learning physiologic principles of tissue salvation through weak supervision. They introduced clinical expert knowledge, built a multiscale CNN (U-Net) together with a convolutional autoencoder and then predicted lesion tissue probabilities for new patients. This approach can predict time-dependent growth of stroke lesions on acute perfusion data, yielding a Dice score overlap of 0.46.[57]

AI-based tissue outcome prediction also has been used in a clinical trial, Eric Acute Stroke Recanalization (ERASER).[59] This trial proposed virtual comparators to investigate whether next-generation mechanical thrombectomy devices can improve outcomes in patients with AIS. The features were extracted from CTP imaging data, enriched by clinical data, and then trained with an RF classifier to generate a predictive model. This model can generate a predictive infarct volume as if a patient received intravenous tissue plasminogen activator therapy. The study showed that the mechanical thrombectomy method led to smaller actual infarct volumes compared the predicted infarct volumes. The highly informative novel study design with virtual comparisons is promising, quick, and relatively inexpensive. The credibility of such trials, however, still needs to be validated.[59]

Many other studies are focused on MRI perfusion-weighted imaging. Ho[63] proposed to train a deep CNN with information from magnetic resonance (MR) perfusion source images to improve tissue outcome prediction and achieved an AUC of 0.87. When compared with other tissue fate models, such as generalized linear model, SVM, and spectral regression and kernel discriminant

analysis, deep CNN proved to be the best model for predicting tissue outcome.[63] Other AI methods have also been applied to MRI imaging. For instance, Giacalone and colleagues[61] applied SVM and Livne and colleagues[62] applied the extreme gradient boosting (XGB) algorithm for MRI-based infarct volume prediction, whereas both studies suggested the role of perfusion parameters as important biomarker for infarct prediction.

One issue with the many algorithms proposed over the recent years is that each of them was developed from separate data sets, and it is difficult to perform head-to-head comparisons among them. The Ischemic Stroke Lesion Segmentation (ISLES) challenge, which has run consecutively for 3 years, aims at addressing this issue of comparability. Using the same data set, multiple teams apply their ML/DL architectures to imaging data in order to make their prediction. Consequently, the performance of their algorithms is compared. In 2015, it was composed of 2 subchallenges: sub-acute stroke lesion segmentation (SISS) and stroke perfusion estimation (SPES). SPES was found to be quite successful, but algorithms applied to subacute lesion segmentation in SISS still lack accuracy.[36] ISLES 2016 and 2017 were focusing on lesion outcome prediction after AIS, using multimodal MRI, including perfusion and diffusion parameters. In ISLES 2016, the results suggested that DL models outperformed RF. CNN-based approaches tended to overestimate lesion segmentation. In ISLES 2017, all participating teams proposed a DL approach with top ranked methods featuring CNN architectures.[67] According to the evolution of methodology over the past years, although further diverse challenges still need to test more models, DL methods, as a variation of CNNs, have set new state-of-the-art benchmarks in many disciplines.

Despite the increased size of training data and different AI architectures used in ISLES 2017, lesion outcome prediction remains a challenge, and there has been minimal improvement compared with ISLES 2016. This observation suggests that CNNs' performance has reached a plateau and other strategies are needed. The ensemble approaches tend to perform better than single models. Pinto and colleagues combined a U-net with a 2-dimensional (2-D) gated recurrent unit layer to obtain smoother and more structured predictions. They also introduced a combination of multimodal MRI maps with nonimaging clinical metadata into an end-to-end DL architecture.[64] By merging imaging with nonimaging clinical information, they tried to obtain a model aware of the principal and collateral blood flow dynamics. Using the ISLES

2017 testing data set, this proposal reached competitive results with a Dice score of approximately 0.29. The investigators admitted, however, that their model still was underperforming expert radiologists, which had a Dice score of 0.58, and additional clinical information may need to be added.

Prediction of Clinical Outcomes

Although many studies are focusing on the prediction of tissue fate, the prediction of future clinical outcomes may be even more useful. Because clinical outcome is a reliable ground-truth, it is an appropriate gold standard in the application of AI to multiple medical conditions. Two different approaches have been proposed to predict clinical outcome based on stroke imaging. The first approach uses quantitative information derived from stroke imaging to perform the prediction. For example, Xie and colleagues[81] proposed XGB and gradient boosting machine (GBM) models to predict modified Rankin scale scores at 90 days, which is the most commonly used outcome measure in studies of these patients. In this study, ASPECTS score, collateral flow score, infarct volume, penumbra volume, and other variables derived from CT images were combined with clinical data to predict the clinical outcome. The results indicated that decision tree–based GBMs can predict the recovery outcome of stroke patients at admission with a high AUC.[81] Another similar approach is by van Os and colleagues,[82] who used multiple ML algorithms to predict the outcome of endovascular treatment of AIS and compared their predictive values. The second approach consists of using stroke imaging directly, with/without clinical data, to perform the prediction. For such an approach, DL algorithms, such as CNN, have been widely used. Generally, 2-D–CNN is applied to the prediction involving 2-D images, and 3-D–CNN is applied to the prediction based on CT, MRI, or videos. Bacchi and colleagues combined a 3-D–CNN for CT-based classification and an ANN for clinical based classification in order to predict clinical outcomes and compared their performances with other methods. Their findings indicated that a combination of CNN and ANN, that is, including both, imaging and clinic information to the model, has the best performance.[82] The prediction of other outcome measures, such as cognitive performance[66] and hemorrhagic transformation after thrombolysis,[56] also has been investigated. For instance, Bentley and colleagues[56] applied different methods for prediction of symptomatic ICH on CT images after thrombolysis, with automatic SVM having the best performance if compared with other prognostic methods, with an AUC of 0.744.

SUMMARY: PERSPECTIVES OF ARTIFICIAL INTELLIGENCE AND STROKE IMAGING

AI has become increasingly ubiquitous in everyday lives. The use of AI in stroke imaging has the potential to detect brain lesions that are barely visible to the naked eye, to improve radiologists' decision making in order to decrease delay to treatment, and to predict patients' clinical outcome.

The ethical and moral concerns with regard to the implementation of AI in clinical diagnostic processes, such as safety, privacy, and bias, are actively discussed.[2,4,5,8,9,11,13,71,83,84] First, AI systems are achieving better performances at the cost of becoming increasingly complex and less interpretable, similar to black boxes. This may cause some distrust from end users toward the applied algorithms. Second, there is a large panel of algorithms/methods to choose from. The performance of models depends not only on the used algorithm but also on the data set used to train, test, and validate them. Current AI is unlike human intelligence in many ways. AI is an advanced statistical method/algorithm based on powerful computing power and massive training data. Current AI, however, can perform only 1 task at a time. Currently, narrow, task-specific AI may match or exceed human performance but still not in complex tasks. For example, despite CNN successes in natural image categorization, it cannot solve any other visual tasks related to many cognitive processing like attention, memory, and executive control. AI can be a good tool to free humans from repetitive and laborious processes of mechanical thinking, similar to going from hand production methods to machines in the first industrial revolution. Much higher levels of AI with top-down knowledge, capability of making associations, or even creative thinking, are needed in the future in order to perform more complex and higher-level tasks.

In conclusion, there is an important need to rapidly and precisely interpret neuroimaging data in stroke, with many potential AI applications. Although AI has the potential to help neuroradiologists, more standardized imaging data sets and more extensive AI studies are needed to establish and validate the role of AI in stroke imaging.

DISCLOSURE

G. Zahachuk and M. Wintermark own equity interest in Subtle Medical.

REFERENCES

1. Lundervold AS, Lundervold A. An overview of deep learning in medical imaging focusing on MRI. Z Med Phys 2019;29:102–27.
2. Suri JS. State-of-the-art review on deep learning in medical imaging. Front Biosci 2018;24:392–426.
3. Maier A, Syben C, Lasser T, et al. A gentle introduction to deep learning in medical image processing. Z Med Phys 2019;29:86–101.
4. Litjens G, Kooi T, Bejnordi BE, et al. A survey on deep learning in medical image analysis. Med Image Anal 2017;42:60–88.
5. Mayo RC, Leung J. Artificial intelligence and deep learning – Radiology's next frontier? Clin Imaging 2018;49:87–8.
6. Fazal MI, Patel ME, Tye J, et al. The past, present and future role of artificial intelligence in imaging. Eur J Radiol 2018;105:246–50.
7. Hosny A, Parmar C, Quackenbush J, et al. Artificial intelligence in radiology. Nat Rev Cancer 2018;18:500–10. Available at: http://www.nature.com/articles/s41568-018-0016-5. Accessed November 30, 2018.
8. Zhu G, Jiang B, Tong L, et al. Applications of Deep Learning to Neuro-Imaging Techniques. Front Neurol 2019;10:1–13.
9. Patel UK, Anwar A, Saleem S, et al. Artificial intelligence as an emerging technology in the current care of neurological disorders. J Neurol 2019. https://doi.org/10.1007/s00415-019-09518-3. Available at: http://www.ncbi.nlm.nih.gov/pubmed/31451912.
10. Sakai K, Yamada K. Machine learning studies on major brain diseases: 5-year trends of 2014–2018. Jpn J Radiol 2019;37:34–72.
11. Zaharchuk G, Gong E, Wintermark M, et al. Deep learning in neuroradiology. AJNR Am J Neuroradiol 2018;39:1776–84. Available at: http://www.ncbi.nlm.nih.gov/pubmed/29419402.
12. Davatzikos C. Machine learning in neuroimaging: Progress and challenges. Neuroimage 2018;197:652–6. Available at: https://linkinghub.elsevier.com/retrieve/pii/S1053811918319621. Accessed November 6, 2018.
13. Gupta MK. Artificial intelligence in diagnosis and management of ischemic stroke. Biomed J Sci Tech Res 2019;13:9964–7.
14. Liebeskind DS. Artificial intelligence in stroke care: Deep learning or superficial insight? EBioMedicine 2018;35:14–5.
15. Kamal H, Lopez V, Sheth SA. Machine learning in acute ischemic stroke neuroimaging. Front Neurol 2018;9:7–12. Available at: https://www.frontiersin.org/article/10.3389/fneur.2018.00945/full.
16. Lee E-J, Kim Y-H, Kim N, et al. Deep into the brain: artificial intelligence in stroke imaging. J Stroke 2017;19:277–85. Available at: http://j-stroke.org/journal/view.php?doi=10.5853/jos.2017.02054. Accessed November 6, 2018.
17. Feng R, Badgeley M, Mocco J, et al. Deep learning guided stroke management: a review of clinical applications. J Neurointerv Surg 2018;10:358–62. Available at: http://jnis.bmj.com/lookup/doi/10.1136/neurintsurg-2017-013355. Accessed November 6, 2018.
18. FDA approves stroke-detecting AI software. Nat Biotechnol 2018;36:290.
19. US Food and Drug Administration. DEN170073 Viz.AI. 2018;90:1–22. Available at: https://www.accessdata.fda.gov/cdrh_docs/reviews/DEN170073.pdf. Accessed September 26, 2019.
20. Ulas C, Das D, Thrippleton MJ, et al. Parameters: Application to stroke dynamic contrast-enhanced MRI. Front Neurol 2019;10:1–14.
21. Kim KH, Choi SH, Park S-H. Improving arterial spin labeling by using deep learning. Radiology 2018;287:658–66. Available at: http://pubs.rsna.org/doi/10.1148/radiol.2017171154.
22. Gibbons EK, Hodgson KK, Chaudhari AS, et al. Simultaneous NODDI and GFA parameter map generation from subsampled q-space imaging using deep learning. Magn Reson Med 2019;81:2399–411.
23. Herweh C, Ringleb PA, Rauch G, et al. Performance of e-ASPECTS software in comparison to that of stroke physicians on assessing CT scans of acute ischemic stroke patients. Int J Stroke 2016;11:438–45.
24. Nagel S, Sinha D, Day D, et al. e-ASPECTS software is non-inferior to neuroradiologists in applying the ASPECT score to computed tomography scans of acute ischemic stroke patients. Int J Stroke 2017;12:615–22. Available at: http://journals.sagepub.com/doi/full/10.1177/1747493016681020. Accessed Novemeber 6, 2018.
25. Gao XW, Hui R, Tian Z. Classification of CT brain images based on deep learning networks. Comput Methods Programs Biomed 2017;138:49–56.
26. Prevedello LM, Erdal BS, Ryu JL, et al. Automated critical test findings identification and online notification system using artificial intelligence in imaging. Radiology 2017;285:923–31. Available at: http://pubs.rsna.org/doi/10.1148/radiol.2017162664. Accessed November 6, 2018.
27. Chilamkurthy S, Ghosh R, Tanamala S, et al. Deep learning algorithms for detection of critical findings in head CT scans: a retrospective study. Lancet 2018;392(10162):2388–96. Available at: https://linkinghub.elsevier.com/retrieve/pii/S0140673618316453. Accessed November 5, 2018.
28. Titano JJ, Badgeley M, Schefflein J, et al. Automated deep-neural-network surveillance of cranial images for acute neurologic events. Nat Med 2018;24:1337–41.

29. Guberina N, Dietrich U, Radbruch A, et al. Detection of early infarction signs with machine learning-based diagnosis by means of the Alberta Stroke Program Early CT score (ASPECTS) in the clinical routine. Neuroradiology 2018;60:889–901. Available at: http://link.springer.com/10.1007/s00234-018-2066-5. Accessed November 6, 2018.

30. Grunwald IQ, Kulikovski J, Reith W, et al. Collateral automation for triage in stroke: evaluating automated scoring of collaterals in acute stroke on computed tomography scans. Cerebrovasc Dis 2019;47(5–6): 217–22.

31. Kuang H, Najm M, Chakraborty D, et al. Automated aspects on noncontrast CT scans in patients with acute ischemic stroke using machine learning. Am J Neuroradiol 2019;40:33–8.

32. Cho J, Park KS, Karki M, et al. Improving sensitivity on identification and delineation of intracranial hemorrhage lesion using cascaded deep learning models. J Digit Imaging 2019;32:450–61.

33. Öman O, Mäkelä T, Salli E, et al. 3D convolutional neural networks applied to CT angiography in the detection of acute ischemic stroke. Eur Radiol Exp 2019;3:8.

34. Score ECT, Albers GW, Wald MJ, et al. Automated calculation of alberta stroke program early CT Score. Stroke 2019;50(11):3277–9.

35. Vincent N, Stier N, Yu S, et al. Detection of hyperperfusion on arterial spin labeling using deep learning. 2015 IEEE International Conference on Bioinformatics and Biomedicine (BIBM). Washington, DC, November 9-12, 2015.

36. Maier O, Menze BH, von der Gablentz J, et al. ISLES 2015 - A public evaluation benchmark for ischemic stroke lesion segmentation from multispectral MRI. Med Image Anal 2017;35:250–69.

37. Kamnitsas K, Ledig C, Newcombe VFJ, et al. Efficient multi-scale 3D CNN with fully connected CRF for accurate brain lesion segmentation. Med Image Anal 2017; 36:61–78. Available at: https://linkinghub.elsevier.com/retrieve/pii/S1361841516301839. Accessed November 5, 2018.

38. Praveen GB, Agrawal A, Sundaram P, et al. Ischemic stroke lesion segmentation using stacked sparse autoencoder. Comput Biol Med 2018;99: 38–52.

39. Pereira S, Meier R, McKinley R, et al. Enhancing interpretability of automatically extracted machine learning features: application to a RBM-Random Forest system on brain lesion segmentation. Med Image Anal 2018;44:228–44. Available at: https://linkinghub.elsevier.com/retrieve/pii/S1361841517301901. Accessed November 6, 2018.

40. Boldsen JK, Engedal TS, Pedraza S, et al. Better diffusion segmentation in acute ischemic stroke through automatic tree learning anomaly segmentation. Front Neuroinform 2018;12:21. http://journal.frontiersin.org/article/10.3389/fninf.2018.00021/full. Accessed November 5, 2018.

41. Ortiz-Ramón R, Valdés Hernández M del C, González-Castro V, et al. Identification of the presence of ischaemic stroke lesions by means of texture analysis on brain magnetic resonance images. Comput Med Imaging Graph 2019;74:12–24.

42. Ho KC, Speier W, Zhang H, et al. A machine learning approach for classifying ischemic stroke onset time from imaging. IEEE Trans Med Imaging 2019;38: 1666–76.

43. Kim C, Zhu V, Obeid J, et al. Natural language processing and machine learning algorithm to identify brain MRI reports with acute ischemic stroke. PLoS One 2019;14:1–13.

44. Chung JW, Kim YC, Cha J, et al. Characterization of clot composition in acute cerebral infarct using machine learning techniques. Ann Clin Transl Neurol 2019;6:739–47.

45. Liu S, Utriainen D, Chai C, et al. Cerebral microbleed detection using Susceptibility Weighted Imaging and deep learning. Neuroimage 2019;198: 271–82.

46. Schirmer MD, Dalca AV, Sridharan R, et al. White matter hyperintensity quantification in large-scale clinical acute ischemic stroke cohorts – The MRI-GENIE study. Neuroimage Clin 2019;23:101884.

47. Livne M, Rieger J, Aydin OU, et al. A U-net deep learning framework for high performance vessel segmentation in patients with cerebrovascular disease. Front Neurosci 2019;13:1–13.

48. Pszczolkowski S, Law ZK, Gallagher RG, et al. Automated segmentation of haematoma and perihaematomal oedema in MRI of acute spontaneous intracerebral haemorrhage. Comput Biol Med 2019;106:126–39.

49. Wu O, Winzeck S, Giese AK, et al. Big data approaches to phenotyping acute ischemic stroke using automated lesion segmentation of multi-center magnetic resonance imaging data. Stroke 2019;50: 1734–41.

50. Kim YC, Lee JE, Yu I, et al. Evaluation of diffusion lesion volume measurements in acute ischemic stroke using encoder-decoder convolutional network. Stroke 2019;50:1444–51.

51. Duong MT, Rudie JD, Wang J, et al. Convolutional neural network for automated FLAIR lesion segmentation on clinical brain MR imaging. Am J Neuroradiol 2019;40:1282–90.

52. Araki T, Jain PK, Suri HS, et al. Stroke risk stratification and its validation using ultrasonic echolucent carotid wall plaque morphology: a machine learning paradigm. Comput Biol Med 2017;80:77–96.

53. Biswas M, Kuppili V, Araki T, et al. Deep learning strategy for accurate carotid intima-media

thickness measurement: An ultrasound study on Japanese diabetic cohort. Comput Biol Med 2018;98:100–17.

54. Biswas M, Kuppili V, Saba L, et al. Deep learning fully convolution network for lumen characterization in diabetic patients using carotid ultrasound: a tool for stroke risk. Med Biol Eng Comput 2019;57:543–64.

55. Zhou R, Fenster A, Xia Y, et al. Deep learning-based carotid media-adventitia and lumen-intima boundary segmentation from three-dimensional ultrasound images. Med Phys 2019;46:3180–93.

56. Bentley P, Ganesalingam J, Carlton Jones AL, et al. Prediction of stroke thrombolysis outcome using CT brain machine learning. Neuroimage Clin 2014;4: 635–40.

57. Lucas C, Kemmling A, Bouteldja N, et al. Learning to predict ischemic stroke growth on acute CT perfusion data by interpolating low -dimensional shape representations. Front Neurol 2018;9:1–15.

58. Kasasbeh AS, Christensen S, Parsons MW, et al. Artificial Neural Network Computer Tomography Perfusion Prediction of Ischemic Core. Stroke 2019;50:1578–81.

59. Fiehler J, Thomalla G, Bernhardt M, et al. Eraser. Stroke 2019;50:1275–8.

60. Bacchi S, Zerner T, Oakden-Rayner L, et al. Deep learning in the prediction of ischaemic stroke thrombolysis functional outcomes: a pilot study. Acad Radiol 2019;27(2):e19–23.

61. Giacalone M, Rasti P, Debs N, et al. Local spatiotemporal encoding of raw perfusion MRI for the prediction of final lesion in stroke. Med Image Anal 2018;50:117–26. Available at: https://linkinghub. elsevier.com/retrieve/pii/S1361841518306807. Accessed November 6, 2018.

62. Livne M, Boldsen JK, Mikkelsen IK, et al. Boosted tree model reforms multimodal magnetic resonance imaging infarct prediction in acute stroke. Stroke 2018;49:912–8. Available at: https://www. ahajournals.org/doi/10.1161/STROKEAHA.117. 019440. Accessed November 6, 2018.

63. Ho KC. Predicting ischemic stroke tissue fate using a deep convolutional neural network on source magnetic resonance perfusion images. J Med Imaging 2019;6:1.

64. Pinto A, Mckinley R, Alves V, et al. Stroke lesion outcome prediction based on MRI imaging combined with clinical information. Front Neurol 2018;9:1–10.

65. Moulton E, Valabregue R, Lehéricy S, et al. Multivariate prediction of functional outcome using lesion topography characterized by acute diffusion tensor imaging. Neuroimage Clin 2019;23:101821.

66. Chauhan S, Vig L, De Filippo De Grazia M, et al. A comparison of shallow and deep learning methods for predicting cognitive performance of stroke patients from MRI lesion images. Front Neuroinform 2019;13:1–12.

67. Winzeck S, Hakim A, McKinley R, et al. ISLES 2016 and 2017-benchmarking ischemic stroke lesion outcome prediction based on multispectral MRI. Front Neurol 2018;9:679. Available at: https://www. frontiersin.org/article/10.3389/fneur.2018.00679/full.

68. Yang Q, Yan P, Zhang Y, et al. Low-dose CT image denoising using a generative adversarial network with wasserstein distance and perceptual loss. IEEE Trans Med Imaging 2018;37:1348–57.

69. Chen KT, Gong E, Bezerra F, et al. Ultra – low-dose 18 F-florbetaben amyloid PET imaging using deep learning with multi-contrast MRI inputs. Radiology 2019;290:649–56.

70. Kassner A, Mandell DM, Mikulis DJ. Measuring permeability in acute ischemic stroke. Neuroimaging Clin N Am 2011;21:315–25, x–xi. Available at: http://www.ncbi.nlm.nih.gov/pubmed/21640302. Accessed September 23, 2013.

71. Mokli Y, Pfaff J, dos Santos DP, et al. Computer-aided imaging analysis in acute ischemic stroke – background and clinical applications. Neurol Res Pract 2019;1:23. Available at: https://neurolrespract.biomedcentral.com/ articles/10.1186/s42466-019-0028-y.

72. Goldenberg R, Peled N. Computer-aided simple triage. Int J Comput Assist Radiol Surg 2011;6:705–11.

73. Thomalla G, Cheng B, Ebinger M, et al. DWI-FLAIR mismatch for the identification of patients with acute ischaemic stroke within 4·5 h of symptom onset (PRE-FLAIR): A multicentre observational study. Lancet Neurol 2011;10:978–86.

74. Emeriau S, Serre I, Toubas O, et al. Can diffusion-weighted imaging-fluid-attenuated inversion recovery mismatch (positive diffusion-weighted imaging/ negative fluid-attenuated inversion recovery) at 3 tesla identify patients with stroke at <4.5 hours? Stroke 2013;44:1647–51.

75. Takahashi N, Lee Y, Tsai DY, et al. An automated detection method for the MCA dot sign of acute stroke in unenhanced CT. Radiol Phys Technol 2014;7:79–88.

76. Dou Q, Chen H, Yu L, et al. Automatic detection of cerebral microbleeds from MR images via 3D convolutional neural networks. IEEE Trans Med Imaging 2016;35:1182–95.

77. Mitra J, Bourgeat P, Fripp J, et al. Lesion segmentation from multimodal MRI using random forest following ischemic stroke. Neuroimage 2014;98: 324–35.

78. Wilke M, de Haan B, Juenger H, et al. Manual, semi-automated, and automated delineation of chronic brain lesions: a comparison of methods. Neuroimage 2011;56:2038–46.

79. Maier O, Schröder C, Forkert ND, et al. Classifiers for ischemic stroke lesion segmentation: a comparison study. PLoS One 2015;10:e0145118. Available at: https://dx.plos.org/10.1371/journal.pone.0145118. Accessed November 5, 2018.

80. Muschelli J, Sweeney EM, Ullman NL, et al. PItcH-PERFeCT: primary intracranial hemorrhage probability estimation using random forests on CT. Neuroimage Clin 2017;14:379–90.

81. Xie Y, Jiang B, Gong E, et al. Use of gradient boosting machine learning to predict patient outcome in acute ischemic stroke on the basis of imaging, demographic, and clinical information. Am J Roentgenol 2019;212:44–51.

82. van Os HJA, Ramos LA, Hilbert A, et al. Predicting outcome of endovascular treatment for acute ischemic stroke: Potential value of machine learning algorithms. Front Neurol 2018;9:1–8.

83. Serre T. Deep learning: the good , the bad , and the ugly. Annu Rev Vis Sci 2019;5:399–426.

84. Saba L, Biswas M, Kuppili V, et al. The present and future of deep learning in radiology. Eur J Radiol 2019;114:14–24.

Updates on Deep Learning and Glioma
Use of Convolutional Neural Networks to Image Glioma Heterogeneity

Daniel S. Chow, MD[a], Deepak Khatri, MD[b], Peter D. Chang, MD[a],
Avraham Zlochower, MD[c], John A. Boockvar, MD[b],
Christopher G. Filippi, MD[c],*

KEYWORDS

• Glioblastoma multiforme • Brain tumor • Deep learning • Convolutional neural networks

KEY POINTS

- Conceptualize how deep learning, as an artificial intelligence (AI) tool, differs from machine learning.
- Review how key genetic mutations in glioma, specifically IDH, EGFR, 1p19q codeletion, and MGMT, are important in diagnosis, treatment planning, and patient management.
- Learn how deep learning algorithms applied to MR imaging can predict genetic status of gliomas and potentially treatment response and survival.

BACKGROUND

Magnetic resonance (MR) imaging is critically important in the diagnosis and treatment management of patients with World Health Organization (WHO) grade IV glioblastoma multiforme (GBM), which remains the most common primary malignant brain tumor. Standard therapy remains the Stupp protocol[1] with maximal surgical resection followed by chemoradiation (temozolomide and radiation therapy). With recurrent glioblastoma, treatment options are limited and narrowed to reresection, antiangiogenic therapy with bevacizumab (Avastin), or clinical trials. Recently, novel treatment strategies in GBM management have included the use of selective intra-arterial delivery of chemotherapeutic agents after blood-brain barrier disruption,[2–4] mesenchymal stem cells for delivery of oncolytic viral agent Delta-24-RGD,[5] a portable, wearable Optune device for tumor-treating fields,[6] intraoperative radiotherapy to the surgical cavity,[7] and chimeric antigen receptor T cells.[8] Despite hundreds of active clinical trials, the prognosis for patients diagnosed with GBM remains dismal, with median survival of 18 to 24 months.[9] Many factors pose significant hurdles to targeted therapeutic approaches in GBM, which lead to their failure, including the intrinsic aggressive nature of a high-grade neoplasm, presence of a perivascular niche of so-called persistor cancer cells,[10] inability of chemotherapeutic agents to efficiently transit the blood-brain barrier effectively, and intrinsic genetic heterogeneity of glioma. With the WHO modifications in 2016 to the classification of gliomas,[11] genetic and molecular information of gliomas is now a critical feature in histopathologic diagnosis.

Renewed interest in the correlation of MR imaging findings to genomics will be challenged by the marked heterogeneity of gliomas. Studies have shown that, within an individual high-grade glial tumor, there is intratumoral variability with

a Department of Radiology, University of California-Irvine School of Medicine, Center for Artificial Intelligence in Diagnostic Medicine (CAIDM), 1001 Health Sciences Road, Orange, CA 92617, USA; b Department of Neurosurgery, Lenox Hill Hospital, Donald and Barbara Zucker School of Medicine at Hofstra/Northwell, 100 East 77th Street, New York, NY 10075, USA; c Department of Radiology, Lenox Hill Hospital, Donald and Barbara Zucker School of Medicine at Hofstra/Northwell, 100 East 77th Street, New York, NY 10075, USA
* Corresponding author.
E-mail address: cfilippi@northwell.edu

Neuroimag Clin N Am 30 (2020) 493–503
https://doi.org/10.1016/j.nic.2020.07.002
1052-5149/20/© 2020 Elsevier Inc. All rights reserved.

different portions of the tumor expressing different genes.[12,13] Thus, any GBM may express different proteins in different areas so a treatment targeted to a particular mutation may only be partially effective despite the specificity of that treatment. Current therapies are unlikely to fully address lesion heterogeneity; hence, the prognosis will remain poor. An emphasis on the genetics of glioma offers potential new therapeutic targets, but intratumoral variability makes standardization of treatment regimens problematic even as a more precision-medicine approach is adopted to tailor individuals' treatments specifically to the genomic mutations expressed by the tumor. This individualized approach to glioma management will be further challenged by current practices in which standard-of-care biopsy and surgical resection samples that undergo pathologic analysis are often incomplete and may not accurately depict the tumor microenvironment. Thus, important genetic features may not be available to neuro-oncologists and neurosurgeons at a time when patients are undergoing treatment and are eligible for clinical trials.

With the emergence of artificial intelligence (AI) in radiology, there is great interest in harnessing the power of MR imaging, which is inherently quantitative, to noninvasively identify the clinical and genetic features of glioma on routine and advanced MR imaging. AI, and more specifically machine learning, which includes deep learning, have the potential to detect patterns in images that remain elusive to the eyes of neuroradiologists, and make predictions with respect to glioma genetics, treatment response, and long-term outcome that can potentially surpass human-level performance. Theoretically, this may enable neuroradiologists to provide greater value to neuro-oncologists and neurosurgeons by providing important information to expedite treatment care that is not currently possible. Prediction of genetic features of glioma from routine MR imaging would also be cost-effective given how widely available MR is as opposed to genomic sequencing, and it is noninvasive.

Deep learning represents end-to-end machine learning in which the process of feature selection from images and classification happen concurrently in one algorithm, and this has the potential to obviate human intervention during training if successfully designed for whole-image analysis. Convolutional neural networks (CNNs) have consistently outperformed and surpassed other competitors in image-related classification tasks, such as the ImageNet competitions where CNNs learn to correctly classify animals and objects.[14–17] Error rates in the ImageNet competitions have continued to decline since 2012 with the use of the AlexNet and currently surpass human-level performance,[14–17] which partly explains the current popularity of CNNs and the shift away from more traditional machine learning approaches. Every MR image has many voxels, all of which contain quantitative information from relaxometry metrics on T1 and T2, apparent diffusion coefficient (ADC) values on diffusion MR, to regional cerebral blood volume (rCBV) on MR perfusion, so extracting this information into a mathematical construct that would allow prediction of genetic markers is the ultimate big data problem for which CNNs may be ideally suited. Unlike classic machine learning, which learns from the examples it receives without explicit programming but often using handcrafted features, a CNN gets input and independently learns on its own the salient features without receiving an explicit example. Given a sufficient quantity of data, CNNs self-interpret, learn, and determine the optimal radiologic features and their relative importance to make a predictive model that can classify an image.[9] The development of CNNs that can accurately predict the status of 1p19q codeletion, isocitrate dehydrogenase (IDH) 1 mutation, EFGR amplification, and MGMT (O-6-methylguanine-DNA-methyltransferease) promoters in glioma have the potential to be a game changer because it may accelerate treatment planning, optimize management, and provide a cheaper and more efficient alternative to expensive genomic sequencing that is not widely available.

ISOCITRATE DEHYDROGENASE MUTATIONS

In the new 2016 WHO classification system, both low-grade astrocytomas and oligodendrogliomas are classified by the presence of IDH1 and IDH2 mutations as well as loss of portions of chromosomes 1 and 19, known as 1p19q codeletion.[11] IDH is an enzyme of the Krebs cycle, which is part of the tumor's metabolic pathway. Normally with IDH wild-type gliomas, there is an accumulation of alpha-ketoglutarate from isocitrate but, with IDH mutations, the isocitrate becomes 2-hydroxyglutarate. Having IDH1 or IDH2 mutations is associated with improved survival,[18] because they respond better to temozolomide therapy. Interestingly, IDH mutations in GBM are most frequently seen in what is considered a secondary GBM when a preexisting low-grade glial tumor evolves into a higher-grade tumor, which confers a better prognosis than IDH wild-type GBM, and these tumors are typically seen in younger patients.[9] Adults diagnosed with IDH wild-type are typically associated with amplification of the EGFRvIII (epidermal growth factor receptor variant III) and the phosphatase and tensin homolog (PTEN) tumor suppressor gene, which results in worse prognosis. IDH mutant gliomas show lower rCBV and flow on MR perfusion and higher ADCs on diffusion MR imaging, which are associated with improved survival.[19–21] Many radiomics studies have had reasonable success correlating MR imaging features with lower-grade gliomas and oligodendrogliomas that express IDH mutations, and these neoplasms have frontal lobe predominance, less or no enhancement, and better delineated tumor margins.[22–24] Furthermore, prediction of IDH mutation status on preoperative MR may improve patient management. A study by Beiko and colleagues[25] reported that resection of nonenhancing tumor after gross total resection of the enhancing component correlated with improvements in progression-free survival in both WHO III and IV gliomas as opposed to IDH wild-type tumors.

Deep learning CNNs, which have done exceptionally well at classification tasks with ImageNet challenges, may be ideally suited to noninvasively predict IDH mutation status of glioma on MR imaging. Yogananda and colleagues[26] developed a three-dimensional (3D) Dense-UNet convolutional neural network trained with 94 cases of IDH mutation and 120 wild-type gliomas from the Tumor Cancer Imaging Archive (TCIA) and The Cancer Genome Atlas (TCGA) using 3-fold cross-validation. The best-performing CNN used multiparametric MR images, achieving 98% sensitivity and 97% specificity, with area under the curve (AUC) of 99%.[26] In an earlier study by Liang and colleagues,[27] they used a multimodal 3D Dense-Net to predict IDH using the publicly available Brain Tumor Imaging Segmentation (BRATS) 2017 database using just 3-T MR scans that included axial T1, postcontrast T1, T2, and fluid-attenuated inversion recovery (FLAIR) images in the model, which came from 102 patients with GBM and 65 patients with low-grade glioma (LGG). This 3D DenseNet model achieved 84.6% accuracy with sensitivity of 78.5%, specificity of 88%, and AUC of 85.7%, but, to obtain optimal model performance, clinical information including age, sex, and tumor grade were included. The lumping of grade III tumors into the LGG category (WHO II) is a limitation to this study.[27] A recent study by Chang and colleagues[28] used a novel two-dimensional (2D)/3D hybrid CNN with 259 cases of LGG and high-grade glioma from the TCIA, achieving an accuracy of 94%. In this article, principal component analysis (PCA) was used to reduce features that were highly correlated with one another in order to determine which features had the largest impact on the final classification

for a particular mutation status.[28] For IDH mutations, the features that mattered most to prediction of IDH mutation status were absent or minimal enhancement, central areas with low T1 and FLAIR signal, and well-defined tumor margins (Fig. 1), whereas the Liang and colleagues[27] article stated that the T2-weighted sequence was the best and nonenhanced T1 the worst for IDH prediction.[28]

Li and colleagues[29] used a deep learning–based radiomics approach to predict IDH1 mutation in a cohort of 151 patients with WHO II LGGs, and the modified CNN had an AUC of 95% when using deep learning–based radiomics on multiple sequences (axial FLAIR and postcontrast T1 MR images) compared with conventional handcrafted radiomics alone (86% AUC). However, this study was limited by lack of independent external validation; use of pathologic diagnoses no longer accepted, such as oligoastrocytoma (30% of cases), and a potential for overfitting given the use of more than 670 features on fewer than 120 tumors with no specific correction mentioned on elimination of redundancy of features in the model.[29] In a multicenter study by Chang and colleagues,[30] a residual convolutional neural network was trained on axial FLAIR, T2, T1 precontrast, and T1 postcontrast images to build a model to predict IDH mutation status in which data augmentation was used to prevent overfitting. Accuracies ranged from 82.8% to 85.7% on the training, validation, and testing models but this improved with the addition of patient age to ranges of 87.3% to 89.1%.[30] A strength of their approach was the use of a logistic regression models based on age with the CNN because IDH mutations are more commonly seen in younger patients with glioma, but limitations to their approach included the absence of more advanced imaging (ADC maps or MR perfusion metrics) and lack of dropout, L1, or L2 regularization that may improve model performance.

1P19Q CODELETION

There is no consensus in the literature for basic noninvasive MR imaging features that can reliably and accurately classify 1p19q codeletion tumors other than a predilection for frontal lobe predominance.[31] These tumors have been reported to be more likely to have indistinct borders, well-defined margins, contrast enhancement, and nonenhancement.[24,31] In a recent study by Ge and colleagues,[32] a novel multistream deep CNN was used to predict 1p19q codeletion status in a cohort of 159 patients using contrast-enhanced T1 MR and T2-weighted MR scans (102 patients with the codeletion and 57 without). The 7-layer 2D CNN used 2D brain image slices to acquire

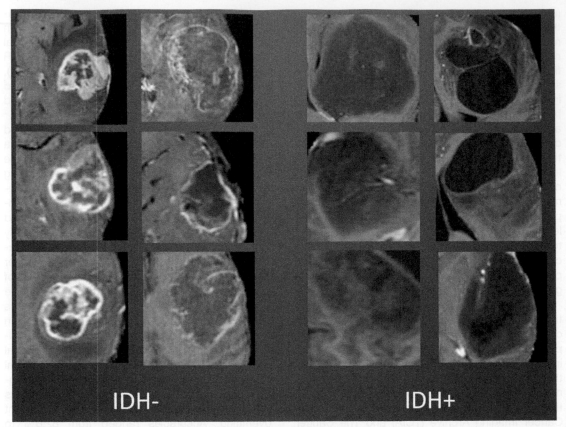

IDH-   IDH+

Fig. 1. 2D-3D hybrid CNN predicting IDH mutation status with 94% accuracy. The 6 images on the left show IDH wild-type and the 6 images on the right show IDH mutation in which the IDH mutation GBMs show minimal or no contrast enhancement, which was determined on PCA to be a key feature that the model used to make its prediction along with well-marginated tumor borders and cysts that were T1 and FLAIR hypointense.

more data, which underwent further data augmentation with 60% of cases for training, 20% for validation, and 20% for holdout, and an accuracy of 89.39% was achieved after 300 epochs of training on the independent dataset.[32] Another study using 159 patients with a multiscale CNN had 87.70% accuracy for prediction of 1p19q codeletion status.[33] In the study by Chang and colleagues,[28] their novel 2D-3D hybrid showed an accuracy of 92% for prediction of 1p19q codeletion status, and they used PCA to reduce features that were highly correlated with one another in order to determine that frontal lobe location, ill-defined tumor borders, and larger amounts of contrast were the most important feature predictors of 1p19q codeletion status[28] (**Fig. 2**).

O-6-METHYLGUANINE-DNA-METHYLTRANSFEREASE PROMOTER

Hypermethylation of MGMT promoter, an enzyme that mediates DNA damage and dealkylates DNA, confers to patients who express this mutation

resistance to the toxicity of temozolomide chemotherapy, which confers a better response and improves prognosis.[34] However, it is also strongly associated with the development of pseudoprogression (PsP) 3 months following chemoradiation after the initial surgery and/or biopsy of the glioma, in which MR images look worse (disease progression) but the patient is responding to therapy.[34–41] Radiomic studies have reported that glial tumors with MGMT promoter mutations have MR features for which reasonable predictions can be made.[28] Chow and colleagues[9] surveyed the literature and also reported that certain semantic or basic quantitative features are associated with MGMT status: MGMT gliomas are less likely to have cystic degeneration and/or necrosis, ring enhancement, solid enhancement, or infiltrative margins,[28–31] whereas these tumors are more likely to have eccentric and/or necrotic cysts, high ADC values, and frontal lobe predominance.[29,30,32,33]

In a study by Han and Kamdar,[42] they used a bidirectional convolutional recurrent neural network architecture developed with Tensorflow

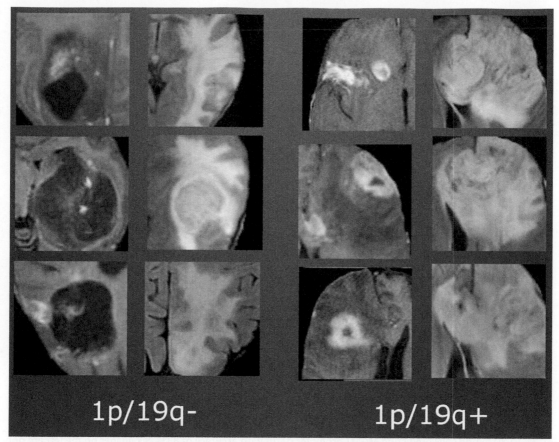

Fig. 2. 2D-3D hybrid CNN predicting 1p19q codeletion status with an accuracy of 92% in which the 6 images on the left show non-1p19q codeletion and the 6 images on the right show 1p19q codeletion. PCA determined that ill-defined tumor margins and greater amounts of enhancement were key imaging features that the CNN used to make its predictions.

Python (https://www.tensorflow.org) on 260 patients acquired from the TCIA and TCGA using T1, T2, and FLAIR scans but no postcontrast T1 scans and obtained an accuracy of 67% on the validation set and 62% on the test data. This study focused on patient-level results in which the predictions were only modestly successful, which may have improved with incorporation of postcontrast images in the training and validation. The unique part of the Han and Kamdar[42] study was the development of an imaging pipeline in which users can choose an individual MR sequence, load it into the CNN interactively, and compare different filters and layers of the model. In earlier work by Levner and colleagues,[43] an artificial neural network was used to predict MGMT promoter in newly diagnosed patients with GBM using features extracted by texture analysis, achieving an accuracy of 87.7% in 59 patients, but only 31 out of 59 had biopsy proof, which is a limitation. In a study by Korfiatis and colleagues,[44] they used and compared 3 different residual CNNs to predict

MGMT status on 155 brain MR examinations with no tumor segmentation preprocessing and achieved accuracies of 94.90%, 80.72%, and 75.75% respectively. In a recent work by Chang and colleagues,[28] using 256 brain MR scans from the TCIA dataset, they had an accuracy of 83% in a 2D-3D hybrid CNN for prediction of the MGMT promoter status that concurrently predicted IDH mutation and 1p19q codeletion status. Using PCA for dimensionality reduction, the study suggested that the most salient features included heterogeneous and nodular enhancement, presence of eccentric cysts, more masslike T2/FLAIR signal with cortical involvement, and slight tendency toward frontal and temporal lobe locations[28] (**Fig. 3**).

EPIDERMAL GROWTH FACTOR RECEPTOR VARIANT III AMPLIFICATION

It is well known that glial tumors with amplification of the EGFRvIII receptor are associated with

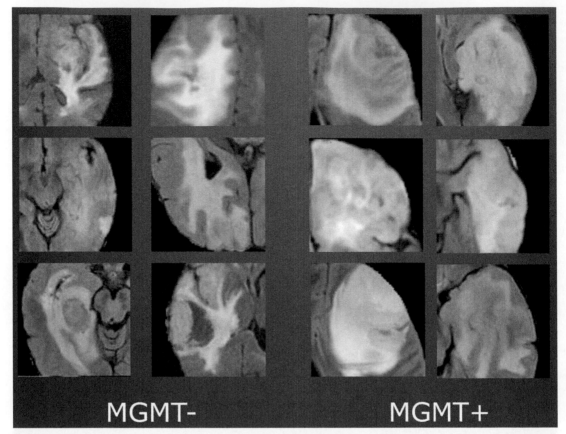

MGMT-   MGMT+

Fig. 3. 2D-3D hybrid CNN predicting MGMT promoter status with accuracy of 83%. Six images on the left are non-MGMT tumors and the 6 on the right have the MGMT promoter. PCA analysis suggested that more heterogeneous enhancement, eccentric cysts, and masslike abnormal T2/FLAIR signal, particularly cortical, were key features used by the CNN to make its model predictions.

angiogenesis promotion, higher cerebral blood volume on MR perfusion, and lower ADC values.[45,46] At present, there are few deep learning AI articles that discuss prediction of epidermal growth factor receptor (EGFR) amplification from preoperative MR images.[47]

PSEUDOPROGRESSION

With the introduction of various therapies, including trails of immunotherapies in GBM management, complex inflammatory responses have emerged, adding to the difficulty in distinguishing PsP from true progression (TP), which remains a diagnostic dilemma in patient management. Many cases of PsP are not reliably diagnosed using response assessment in neuro-oncology (RANO) criteria.[48] A recent meta-analysis suggested that up to 36% of cases are underdiagnosed.[49] Jang and colleagues[50] used a hybrid deep and machine learning CNN-LSTM (long short-term memory) technique on patients with

GBM from a couple of institutions to classify PsP from TP, achieving an AUC of 0.83. In a machine learning study by Akbari and colleagues,[51] a support vector machine (SVM)–based analysis was conducted on conventional and advanced MR imaging features by training the model on pathologists' scores of TP versus PsP and found high correlation ($r = 0.86$) between pathologic and radiomic scores of PsP. To date, there are few deep learning publications addressing PsP, likely related to a lack of ground truth or histopathologically proven cases as well as an insufficient number of well-curated, annotated MR images of PsP cases. At this time, the question of PsP versus TP remains a critical, unmet need.

OVERALL SURVIVAL AFTER DIAGNOSIS WITH GLIOBLASTOMA MULTIFORME

Independent risk factors affect progression-free survival and overall survival (OS) in patients diagnosed with GBM. Male gender, old age at the time of diagnosis (age>60 years), poor preoperative Karnofsky scores of less than 70 (a clinical metric of functional status), advanced tumor with partial resection, and surgery without adjuvant chemoradiation are all associated with worse outcomes,[52,53] and a recent large-scale epidemiologic study suggests that Asian people and Pacific Islanders have better survival compared with white people.[54] In a study by LaCroix and colleagues,[55] they identified 5 independent predictors of OS in patients with GBM, including age, Karnofsky Performance Scale scores, extent of resection, degree of necrosis, and enhancement on preoperative MR imaging. In a prior study by Pope and colleagues,[56] T1 MR features were found to contribute largely to prediction of OS and, among all MR features, both nonenhancing tumor and areas of infiltration were good predictors of OS. Jain and colleagues[57] showed that tumors with higher rCBV in nonenhanced regions on MR dynamic susceptibility perfusion tended to have worse survival, and Jain and colleagues[58] later found that high-grade gliomas with EGFRvIII amplification and high rCBV had worse OS.

In a study by Sun and colleagues,[59] a 3D CNN was used for tumor segmentation followed by an machine learning (ML) program that extracted radiomics features using a decision tree regression model to determine the top-ranked features, which were then used with a random forest model to predict OS in patients with GBM, achieving a modest 61% accuracy on short-term (<10 months), midterm (between 10 and 15 months), and long-term (>15 months) survivors.[59] This study used 210 high-grade gliomas and 75 LGGs from the BRATS 2018 dataset for training and 66 brain tumor cases of unknown grade on the validation set in which FLAIR, T1, T1 postcontrast, and T2 images were used to train the model.[59]

In a study by Nie and colleagues,[60] they used a 3D CNN to automatically extract features from multimodal preoperative brain MR images (T1, functional MR imaging, and diffusion tensor imaging) of high-grade gliomas (69 patients with either WHO III or IV tumors), using multichannel and learning supervised features to train a SVM model to predict long-term versus short-term OS in patients with GBM with greater than 22 months representing long-term survival. In this study, handcrafted features were added to the SVM model, including age at diagnosis, gender, tumor location, tumor size, and WHO grade; greatest accuracy was obtained using a 3D CNN with the SVM and handcrafted features at nearly 90%.[60] Subsequently, this research group applied similar methodology using deep learning CNN to automatically extract high-level features from multimodal, multichannel preoperative MR scans using T1, axial diffusion tensor imaging, and axial resting state connectivity maps (resting state functional MR imaging) from 68 patients with high-grade glioma in which this information, along with selected clinical features, specifically age, tumor size, and histopathologic subtype, were used to train an SVM to predict short-term versus long-term survival in patients with GBM, achieving 90.66% accuracy.[61] Limitations of this work include the lack of independent test sets, MR brain examinations coming from a single institution using the same 3-T MR system from 1 manufacturer, and an arbitrary threshold of 650 days to define good versus poor survival as a binary choice fixed on that time point. The greatest limitation is failure to include genomic data (IDH, EGFR, and MGMT status) and failure to include extent of tumor resection (partial vs gross total resection) as well as the type and duration of treatment, such as chemoradiation versus other treatments. In an abstract by Chang and colleagues,[62] clinical features (tumor location, age, and Karnofsky scores) combined with a 2D-3D hybrid CNN were used to predict good survival (>24 months) and poor survival (<6 months) with 82% accuracy (**Fig. 4**).

CHALLENGES AND THE FUTURE

Routine clinical use of AI algorithms for neuroimaging faces many challenges. The development of AI algorithms is hindered by the need for large datasets that are well annotated. The annotation of images is costly and time consuming because physicians are more valuable, to administrators, reading clinical cases. There need to be automated tools to reduce that burden.

Furthermore, sharing data may require a rethinking of academic medical research practice with a horizontal framework as opposed to the traditional vertical, hierarchical structure. A collective effort by multiple institutions may be required in order to pool data and to compete with private-sector companies that are routinely purchasing large amounts of medical data.

Any CNN may underperform when prospectively tested on external data in real-world situations in health care networks that have multiple different MR vendors and marked heterogeneity in MR imaging protocols. Standardization of imaging protocols may be needed on a large scale to achieve homogeneity of the data, and structured reporting may assist in the scalability of data mining of electronic medical records. Additional challenges include ground-truth genomics for all studies involving CNNs and MR imaging, which is true

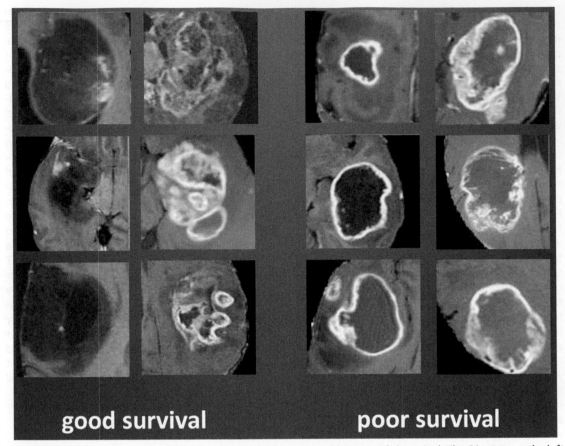

good survival   **poor survival**

Fig. 4. 2D-3D hybrid CNN predicting poor (<6 months) versus good (>24 months) survival. The 6 images on the left were classified as good survival, whereas the 6 images on the right were classified as poor survival with an accuracy of 82% using clinical information in the model (age, tumor location, and Karnofsky scores).

for all of oncologic imaging and not just gliomas. The heterogeneity of glioma, in particular, may necessitate changes in practice, with more sampling and/or biopsies even in cases of gross total resection. In addition, thought needs to be given to how to integrate CNNs into routine workflow (cloud solutions, on-site solutions embedded in Picture archiving and communication system [PACS]) so that the workflow of neuroradiologists is not disrupted. If there are too many mouse clicks, no one will bother to use the deployed algorithm.

Multiple articles have shown that CNNs are clearly doing well at the prediction of IDH mutations and 1p19a codeletions, and reasonably well at MGMT promoter predictions on routine preoperative brain MR studies, although there is still a need for more work on EGFRvIII prediction and PsP prediction. With newer code architecture, more data with ground-truth genomics, and CNNs combined with clinical data, performances are likely to improve. To get full-scale buy-in from neuroradiologists, it is likely that more deep

learning studies will need to engage in techniques that will peer into the "black box" of CNNs, so that neuroradiologists can be informed by the AI algorithm regarding what features were most germane to a particular genomic prediction model. In this way, neuroradiologists will develop augmented intelligence from the AI that they are using, which will enhance the value neuroradiologists provide to the clinical mission of precision patient care.

REFERENCES

1. Stupp R, Mason WP, van der Bent MJ, et al. Radiotherapy plus concomitant and adjuvant temozolomide for glioblastoma. N Engl J Med 2005;352:987–96.
2. Chakraborty S, Filippi CG, Burkhardt JK, et al. Durability of single dose intra-arterial bevacizumab after blood-brain barrier disruption for recurrent glioblastoma. J Exp Ther Oncol 2016;11(4):261–7.
3. Alter RA, White TG, Fanous AA, et al. Long-term benefit of intra-arterial bevacizumab for recurrent glioblastoma. J Exp Ther Oncol 2017;12(1):67–71.

4. Kaluson KO, Schneider JR, Chakraboty S, et al. Superselective intra-arterial cerebral infusion of cetuximab with blood brain barrier disruption combined with stupp protocol for newly diagnosed GBM. J Exp Ther Oncol 2018;12(3): 23–229.

5. Lang FF, Conrad C, Gomez-Manzano C, et al. Phase I study of DNX-2401 (Delta 24-RGD) oncolytic adenovirus: replication and immunotherapeutic effects in recurrent glioblastoma. J Clin Oncol 2018; 36(14):1419–27.

6. Onken J, Staub-Bartelt F, Najkoczy P, et al. Acceptance and compliance of TTFields treatment among high grade glioma patients. J Neurooncol 2018; 139(1):17–184.

7. Straube C, Scherb H, Gempt J, et al. Adjuvant stereotactic fractionated radiotherapy to the resection cavity in recurrent glioblastoma: the GlioCave Study (NOA 17-ARO 2016/3-DKTK ROG Trial). BMC Cancer 2018;18(1):15.

8. Petersen CT, Krenciute G. Next generation CAR T-cells for the immunotherapy of high grade glioma. Front Oncol 2019;9:69.

9. Chow DS, Chang P, Weinberg B, et al. Imaging genetic heterogeneity in glioblastoma. AJR Am J Roentgenol 2018;210(1):30–8.

10. Sattiraju A, Mintz A. Pericytes in glioblastoma: multifaceted role within tumor microenvironments and potential for therapeutic interventions. Adv Exp Med Biol 2019;1147:65–91.

11. Louis DN, Perry A, Reifenberger G, et al. The 2016 World Health Organization classification of tumors of the central nervous system: a summary. Acta Neuropathol 2016;131:803–20.

12. Patel AP, Tirosh I, Trombetta JJ, et al. Single-cell RNA-seq highlights intratumoral heterogeneity of primary glioblastoma. Science 2014;344(6190): 1396–401.

13. Sottoriva A, Spiteri J, Piccirillo SG, et al. Intratumoral heterogeneity in human glioblastoma reflects cancer evolutionary dynamics. Proc Natl Acad Sci U S A 2013;110:4009–14.

14. Le Cun Y, Bengio Y, Hinton G. Deep learning. Nature 2015;521:436–44.

15. Simonyan K, Vedaldi A, Zisserman A. Deep Inside Convolutional Neural Networks: Visualising Image Classification Models and Saliency Maps. Available at: https://arxiv.org/abs/1312.6034. Accessed December 20, 2019.

16. Krizhevsky A, Sutskever I, Hinton G. ImageNet Classification with Deep Convolutional Neural Networks. Abstract in Proceedings of Advances in Neural Information Processing Systems 25 (NIPS 2012). Lake Tahoe (NV), December 3, 2012.

17. He K, Zhang X, Ren S, et al. Deep Residual Learning for Image Recognition. Available at: https://arxiv.org/abs/1512.03385. Accessed December 21, 2019.

18. Ducray F, Idbaih A, Wang XW, et al. Predictive and prognostic factors for glioma. Expert Rev Anticancer Ther 2011;11:781–9.

19. Kickengereder P, Sahm F, Radbruch A, et al. IDH mutation status is associated with a distinct hypoxia/angiogenesis transcriptome which is noninvasively predicable with rCBV imaging in human glioma. Sci Rep 2015;5:16238.

20. Law M, Young RJ, Babb JS, et al. Gliomas: predicting time to progression or survival with cerebral blood volume measurements at dynamic susceptibility-weighted contrast-enhanced perfusion MR imaging. Radiology 2008;247: 490–8.

21. Carillo JA, Lai A, Nghiemphu PL, et al. Relationship between tumor enhancement, edema, IDH1 mutation status, MGMT promoter methylation, and survival in glioblastoma. AJNR Am J Neuroradiol 2012;33:1349–55.

22. Paldor I, Pearce FC, Drummond KJ, et al. Frontal glioblastoma multiforme may be biologically distinct from non-frontal and multilobular tumors. J Clin Neurosci 2016;34:128–32.

23. Sonoda Y, Shibahara I, Kawaguchi T, et al. Association between molecular alterations and tumor location and mri characteristics in anaplastic gliomas. Brain Tumor Pathol 2015;32:99–104.

24. Qi S, Yu L, Li H, et al. Isocitrate dehydrogenase mutation is associated with tumor location and magnetic resonance imaging characteristics in astrocytic neoplasms. Onco Lett 2014;7:1895–902.

25. Beiko J, Suki D, Hess KR, et al. IDH mutant malignant astrocytomas are more amenable to surgical resection and have a survival benefit associated with maximal surgical resection. Neuro Oncol 2014;16:81–91.

26. Yogananda CGB, Shah BR, Vejdani-Jahromi M, et al. A Novel Fully Automated MRI-based Deep Learning Method for Classification of IDH mutation status in brain gliomas. Neuro Oncol 2020;22(3): 402–11.

27. Liang S, Zhang R, Liang D, et al. Multimodal 3D DenseNet for IDH genotype prediction in gliomas. Genes 2018;9:1–17.

28. Chang P, Grinband J, Weinberg BD, et al. Deep learning convolutional neural networks accurately classify genetic mutations in glioma. AJNR Am J Neuroradiol 2018;39(7):1201–7.

29. Li Z, Wang Y, Yu J, et al. Deep learning based radiomics (DLR) and its usage in noninvasive IDH1 prediction for low grade glioma. Sci Rep 2017;7:5467.

30. Chang K, Bai HX, Zhou H, et al. Residual convolutional neural networks for determination of IDH status in low- and high grade gliomas from MR imaging. Clin Cancer Res 2018;24(5):1073–81.

31. Xiong J, Tan W, Wen J, et al. Combination of diffusion tensor imaging and conventional MRI correlates

with isocitrate dehydrogenase1/2 Mutations but Not 1p19q genotyping in oligodendroglial tumors. Eur Radiol 2016;26:1705–15.

32. Ge C, Gu IY, Jakola AS, et al. Deep learning and multi-sensor fusion for glioma classification using multistream 2D convolutional neural networks. Conf Proc IEEE Eng Med Biol Soc 2018;2018: 5894–7.

33. Akkus Z, Ali I, Sedlar J, et al. Predicting deletion of chromosomal arms of 1p/19q in low-grade glioma from MR images using machine intelligence. J Digit Imaging 2017;30(4):469–76.

34. Hegi ME, Diserens AC, Gorlia T, et al. MGMT gene silencing and benefit from temozolomide in glioblastoma. N Engl J Med 2005;352:997–1003.

35. Gorlia T, van den Bent MJ, Hegi ME, et al. Nomograms for predicting survival of patients with newly diagnosed glioblastoma: prognostic factor analysis of EORTC and NCIC Trial 26981-22981/CE.3. Lancet Oncol 2008;9:29–38.

36. Kansas VG, Zacharaki EI, Thomas GA, et al. Learning MRI-based classification models for MGMT methylation status prediction in glioblastoma. Comput Methods Programs Biomed 2017;140: 249–57.

37. Drabycz S, Roldan G, de Robles P, et al. An analysis of image texture, tumor location, and MGMT promoter methylation in glioblastoma using magnetic resonance imaging. Neuroimage 2010;49: 1398–405.

38. Moon WJ, Choi JW, Roh HG, et al. Imaging parameters of high-grade gliomas in relation to the MGMT promoter methylation status: the CT, diffusion tensor, and perfusion MR imaging. Neuroradiology 2012;54: 555–63.

39. Eoli M, Menghi F, Bruzzone MG, et al. Methylation of O6-Methylguanine DNA methyltransferase and loss of heterozygosity on 19q and/or 1p are overlapping features of secondary glioblastoma with prolonged survival. Clin Cancer Res 2007;13: 2606–13.

40. Ellingson BM, Lai A, Harris RJ, et al. Probabilistic radiographic atlas of glioblastoma phenotypes. AJNR Am J Neuroradiol 2013;34:1326–33.

41. Romano A, Calabria LF, Tavanti F, et al. Apparent diffusion coefficient obtained by magnetic resonance imaging as a prognostic marker inglioblastomas: correlation with MGMT promoter methylation status. Eur Radiol 2013;23:513–20.

42. Han L, Kamdar MR. MRI to MGMT: predicting methylation status in glioblastoma using convolutional recurrent neural networks. Pac Symp Biocomput 2018;23:331–42.

43. Levner I, Drabycz S, Roldan G, et al. Predicting MGMT methylation status of glioblastoma from MRI texture. In International Conference of Medical Image Computing and Computer-assisted Intervention-MICCAI. London, September 20, 2009. p. 552-530.

44. Korfiatis P, Kline TL, Lachance DH, et al. Residual deep convolutional neural network predicts MGMT methylation status. J Digit Imaging 2017; 30:622–8.

45. Young RJ, Gupta A, Shah AD, et al. Potential role of preoperative conventional MRI including diffusion measurements in assessing epidermal growth factor receptor gene amplification status in patients with glioblastoma. AJNR Am J Neuroradiol 2013;34: 2271–7.

46. Gupta A, Young RJ, Shah AD, et al. Pretreatment dynamic susceptibility contrast MRI perfusion in glioblastoma: prediction of EGFR gene amplification. Clin Neuroradiol 2015;25:143–50.

47. Hedyehzadeh M, Maghooli K, MomenGharibvand M. A comparison of the efficiency of using a deep CNN approach with other common regression methods for the prediction of EGFR expression in glioblastoma patients. J Digit Imaging 2020;33:391–8.

48. Nasseri M, Gahramanov S, Netto JP, et al. Evaluation of pseudoprogression in patients with glioblastoma multiforme using dynamic magnetic resonance imaging with ferumoxytol calls RANO criteria into question. Neuro Oncol 2014;16: 1146–54.

49. Abbasi AW, Westerlan HE, Holtman GA, et al. Incidence of tumor progression and pseudoprogression in high grade gliomas: a systematic review and meta-analysis. Clin Neuroradiol 2018;28: 401–11.

50. Jang BS, Jeon SH, Kim IH, et al. Predictor of pseudoprogression versus progression using machine learning algorithm in glioblastoma. Sci Rep 2018;8: 12516.

51. Akbari H, Bakas S, Martinez-Lage M, et al. Quantitative radiomics and machine learning to distinguish true progression from pseudoprogression in patients with GBM. Presented at the 56th annual meeting of the American Society for Neuroradiology, Vancouver, BC, Canada, June 2–7, 2018.

52. Wang J, Hu G, Quan X. Analysis of the factors affecting the prognosis of glioblastoma patients. Open Med 2019;14:331–5.

53. Tian M, Ma W, Chen Y, et al. Impact of gender on the survival of patients with glioblastoma. Biosci Rep 2018;38(6):1–9.

54. Thumma SR, Fairbanks RK, Lamoureux WT, et al. Effect of pretreatment clinical factors on overall survival in glioblastoma multiforme: a surveillance epidemiology and end results (SEER) population analysis. World J Surg Oncol 2012; 10:75.

55. LaCroix M, Abi-Said D, Fourney DR, et al. A multivariate analysis of 416 patients with glioblastoma multiforme: prognosis, extent of

resection, and survival. J Neurosurg 2001;95(2): 190–8.

56. Pope WB, Sayre J, Perlina A, et al. MR imaging correlates of survival in patients with high grade glioma. AJNR Am J Neuroradiol 2005;26(10):2466–74.

57. Jain R, Poisson L, Narang J, et al. Genomic mapping and survival prediction in glioblastoma: molecular subclassification strengthened by hemodynamic imaging biomarkers. Radiology 2013;267:212–20.

58. Jain R, Poisson LM, Gutman D, et al. Outcome prediction in patients with glioblastoma by using imaging, clinical, and genomic biomarkers: focus on the nonenhancing component of the tumor. Radiology 2014;272:484–93.

59. Sun L, Zhang S, Chen H, et al. Brain tumor segmentation and survival prediction using multimodal MRI scans with deep learning. Front Neurosci 2019;13:1–8.

60. Nie D, Lu J, Zhang H, et al. Multi-channel 3D deep feature learning for survival time prediction of brain tumor patients using multi-modal neuroimages. Sci Rep 2019;9(1–14):1103.

61. Nie D, Zhang H, Adeli E, et al. 3D deep learning for multi-modal imaging-guided survival time prediction of brain tumor patients. Med Image Comput Assist Interv 2016;9901:212–20.

62. Chang P, Maffie J, Lignelli A, et al. Deep Learning and Glioma Radiogenomics: A TCIA/TCGA Project. Abstract in Proceedings of the Annual American Society of Neuroradiology (ASNR) Meeting. Long Beach (CA); 2017.

Diverse Applications of Artificial Intelligence in Neuroradiology

Michael Tran Duong, BA[a], Andreas M. Rauschecker, MD, PhD[b],
Suyash Mohan, MD[a,*]

KEYWORDS

- Neuroradiology • Artificial intelligence • Deep learning • Neural network • Trauma
- Multiple sclerosis • Epilepsy • Neurodegeneration

KEY POINTS

- Artificial intelligence (AI) has the potential to improve efficiency and accuracy in neuroradiology.
- AI tools are starting to be validated for tasks such as workflow optimization, segmentation, and precision education for a variety of brain diseases.
- Future AI may integrate imaging data with additional diagnostic data from the medical record.

INTRODUCTION

Globally, neurologic and mental disorders affect 1 in 3 people across their lifetime.[1] Uniquely positioned to improve imaging diagnosis and clinical management for patients with brain diseases, artificial intelligence (AI) is a computational model that can parallel human performance on tasks, often without explicit programming. Several classes of AI have been studied extensively, including machine learning (ML) and deep learning (DL), which uses artificial neural networks (NN) inspired by neuronal architectures.[2,3]

Imaging research in AI has grown exponentially. As of 2019, there are approximately 9000 PubMed indexed articles that match the search on AI and imaging/radiology and approximately 5000 articles on AI and neuroimaging/neuroradiology (Fig. 1). Consequently, a thorough discussion on the technology and applications of AI in radiology is beyond the scope of this review and can be found elsewhere.[4-8] Discussion of AI for brain tumor, infarct, and hemorrhage imaging can be found elsewhere in this issue. Because of the ability of NNs to learn any input-output function,[9] whether based on imaging or not, the potential applications of NNs to radiology span not only image-based tasks but also the many non–image-based tasks that radiologists perform.

Here, we overview a diverse array of current neuroimaging applications of AI, including tasks such as worklist prioritization, lesion detection, anatomic segmentation, safety, quality, and precision education, in a diverse set of diseases ranging from neurodegeneration to trauma. Then, we introduce emerging applications, including multimodal integration for neuroradiology. Finally, we discuss challenges and potential solutions for widespread adoption of AI in neuroimaging clinics worldwide.

DIVERSE APPLICATIONS FOR ARTIFICIAL INTELLIGENCE IN NEURORADIOLOGY

Throughout the review, we survey a variety of current and emerging applications for AI, ML, and DL toward a range of neurologic disorders, from

---

[a] Department of Radiology, Perelman School of Medicine at the University of Pennsylvania, 3400 Spruce Street, 219 Dulles Building, Philadelphia, PA 19104, USA; [b] Department of Radiology & Biomedical Imaging, University of California, San Francisco, 513 Parnassus Avenue, Room S-261, San Francisco, CA 94143, USA
* Corresponding author.
E-mail address: suyash.mohan@pennmedicine.upenn.edu
Twitter: @MichaelDuongMD (M.T.D.); @DrDreMDPhD (A.M.R.); @drsuyash (S.M.)

Neuroimag Clin N Am 30 (2020) 505–516
https://doi.org/10.1016/j.nic.2020.07.003

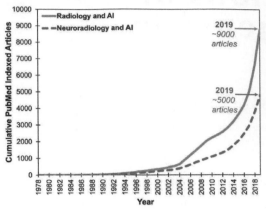

Fig. 1. Cumulative frequency of PubMed indexed articles on AI and imaging/radiology (*gray line*) and AI and neuroimaging/neuroradiology (*blue dashed line*). Boolean search query for radiology was "AI/ML/DL/NN and clinical/medical and imaging/radiology/body" and for neuroradiology was "AI/ML/DL/NN and clinical/medical and neuroimaging/neuroradiology/brain." PubMed last accessed November 27, 2019.

trauma to multiple sclerosis, epilepsy to neurodegeneration. Compared with previous reviews of AI in neuroimaging organized by technical developments and AI methods, this review is organized by clinical tasks relevant to neuroradiology.

Worklist Prioritization

Because of the unique structure, function, and location of the brain, diagnosis of neurologic diseases largely depends on imaging. Time from imaging to proper diagnosis and management can be a determinant of patient outcomes for acute and chronic neurologic diseases.[10–12]

Patients presenting with acute ischemic stroke progress in a sequence from door to imaging to diagnosis and intervention. Shorter door-to-puncture time for intravenous thrombolysis and/or mechanical thrombectomy is associated with better long-term functional outcomes.[13,14] One solution to improve door-to-puncture times and outcomes is to reduce imaging-to-diagnosis time, and this may be implemented with standardized, automated worklist prioritization. Natural language processing (NLP) algorithms and automated lesion detection networks (described in the next section) may augment efficiency in triaging imaging studies of patients with acute, time-sensitive presentations. NLP and NNs have already been applied to interpretation of chest computed tomography (CT) reports[15] and abdominal CT and pathology reports,[16,17] and such tools may be similarly applied to head CT.

Future iterations of such automated detection algorithms may be integrated into radiology workflows to improve efficiency. Indeed, current AI tools on the market can send processed imaging data such as CT perfusion maps via text message to stroke physicians and neurointerventional radiologists in real-time. Further, automated segmentation has been applied to workflow integration for patients presenting with intracranial hemorrhage, and such networks could be applied to all patients with head CTs presenting with acute neurologic deficits.[18] Despite the high accuracies attained by such networks for detecting findings, challenges of integrating these algorithms into the clinical workflow remain. For example, some intracranial hemorrhages are expected (such as after craniotomy), whereas others may be unexpected, and therefore much more urgent. Integrating such clinical context into the prioritization score is essential for ensuring that potentially more urgent studies are not deprioritized.

Worklist prioritization may also improve radiology education. Because radiology trainee performance increases with optimal case exposure and volume,[19] AI may assign specific cases to trainees based on their training profile, to promote consistency in individual trainee experiences.[20]

Lesion Detection

Neurologic diagnoses are made through clinical assessments of patient function and detection and interpretation of lesions on neuroimaging. Furthermore, lesion burden is often associated with functional impairment. Hence, accurate detection and characterization of lesions on neuroimaging is vital to expedite diagnosis and management. Across a variety of brain diseases, there are many research applications for AI in segmentation and quantification of image features.

Trauma

Trauma is a common indication for neuroimaging. DL models such as convolutional neural networks (CNNs) have been designed to detect spinal cord contusion injuries. Demonstrating clinical utility, the quantified injury volumes correlate well with motor impairment.[21] Many methods use CNNs to detect and classify hemorrhages such as epidural and subdural hematomas and subarachnoid and intraparenchymal hemorrhage on head CT scans.[22,23] In addition, ML techniques such as random forest models have been applied to assess white matter hyperintensities in patients with traumatic brain injury.[24]

Metastatic disease

Brain metastases occur in about 20% of patients with cancer. Metastatic disease encompasses a clinically and radiographically heterogeneous set of diseases that often has distinct imaging features and warrants management unique from primary tumors. For example, mucinous metastases can have T2w signal hypointensities, metastatic melanoma can display T1w signal hyperintensities, and metastatic breast cancer can demonstrate necrotic and cystic lesions.[25] Using the brain tumor Segmentation (BraTS) challenge datasets, recent DL methods have assessed metastases in multisequence magnetic resonance (MR) studies, including fluid-attenuated inversion recovery (FLAIR) and pre- and postgadolinium enhanced T1-weighted images.[26–28] Such networks are therefore useful for stereotactic surgical planning.

Multiple sclerosis

Multiple sclerosis (MS) diagnosis and progression depends on neuroimaging, wherein patients present with white matter lesions disseminated over space and time.[29] Hence, AI can be extremely beneficial for the quantification and tracking of specific lesions in individual patients. A variety of research AI models (including NNs, k-nearest neighbors and support vector machines [SVM]) exist for detecting MS lesions with high specificity and sensitivity.[30–32]

Diverse causes

Overall, many pathologies demonstrate hyperintense lesions on FLAIR sequences. Methods exist to segment white matter hyperintensities in diseases such as Alzheimer disease (AD) and small vessel ischemic disease.[33,34] However, in the clinical workflow, the diagnosis that a patient presents with is not always known, and methods are required to recognize abnormalities despite diagnostic uncertainty. Recently, our group has shown that a CNN with U-net architecture can perform at near radiologist-level accuracy for detecting lesions across a variety of pathologies, at fractions of the time.[35] Such general task-specific, rather than disease-specific, approaches have the potential to be applied universally to neuroimaging. Ultimately, such methods may decrease the rate of perceptual errors in neuroradiology, which are the basis of most diagnostic errors.[36,37]

Anatomic Segmentation and Volumetry

Neuroanatomy is variable across individuals and difficult to segment computationally, particularly when anatomy is distorted by underlying pathology. However, AI has made significant inroads in the segmentation and parcellation of cortical and subcortical structures.[38,39] Such anatomic classification AI could be useful for planning stereotactic radiosurgery and surgical resection for pathologies from neoplasia to epileptogenic foci and heterotopias.

Atrophy is essential in diagnosing certain neurodegenerative diseases and AI is well positioned to enable quantification of anatomic changes. CNNs and SVMs can compare volumetrics of different brain regions including the hippocampus in dementia[40–43] and basal ganglia in Huntington disease.[44,45] For white matter diseases, current DL networks can detect and measure abnormalities, including volumetrics.[34,35] In the future, these tools can be combined with enhanced anatomic linking to calculate changes over time.

Patient Safety and Quality Improvement

Protocoling

In addition to diagnosis, patient safety and image quality measures can be improved with AI. The first step of an imaging examination involving a radiologist is often the study protocoling, which can have a major impact on diagnostic accuracy at the time of image interpretation. Methods are being developed for standardizing and improving the protocoling process.[46]

Contrast agents

Contrast agents and radiotracers pose nonzero risks to patients. Recent studies suggest as few as 2 doses of gadolinium-based contrast agents can lead to gadolinium deposition in dentate nuclei, globi pallidi, and other deep brain structures.[47] Accordingly, CNNs may reduce the gadolinium dose required to interpret enhancing lesions on brain MR imaging[48,49] and even radiation exposure on CT.[50,51]

For nuclear medicine studies, DL algorithms are being developed to create "synthetic" amyloid PET to reduce radiotracer volume injected. By training CNNs on PET images with lower signal-to-noise ratios, several studies have predicted how amyloid PET images would appear if the patient were given a full radiotracer dose based on PET images representing much lower (<1%) doses of tracer.[52–55] Additional studies leverage reconstruction PET with generative adversarial networks to promote more rigorous training of AI systems for diverse inputs.[56]

The clinical impact of such approaches remains to be rigorously studied. Although the technical achievements of these dose-reduction algorithms are considerable, the underlying principles of information theory cannot be understated. That is, an AI algorithm cannot create signal if the information is not present in the first place. Although much of

MR image information is redundant, it is likely that in some unexpected cases, the administration of contrast adds information that cannot be gleaned from the remainder of the sequences. To what extent denoising algorithms will provide the correct predictions in these minority cases remains to be seen. Thus, before their clinical implementation, such algorithms must be diligently evaluated across a diverse spectrum of cases in the real clinical workflow.

Image reconstruction

Once raw data are acquired, the information contained in sensor space must be reconstructed into an image. Understanding this process as a function that maps an input (sensor space) to an output (the image) reframes this problem as one that could be solved by an AI algorithm, bypassing traditional reconstruction algorithms including the traditional Fourier transform from K-space. Indeed, the AUTOMAP method was recently developed to perform this mapping.[57] Although promising, such new methods will still need to be evaluated in the context of clinical MR imagings to determine that they do not compromise patient safety.

Recall rates

Proper diagnosis depends on image quality. AI can improve the speed and accuracy of diagnosis by reducing recalls and rescans due to artifacts such as motion. The requisite image quality for different scans depends on the indication and the reading radiologist. Therefore, AI for patient diagnosis should be adapted for each patient and radiologist. Indeed, a recent study demonstrated how DL models can reduce recall and rescan rates for imaging studies of MS and stroke.[58]

Precision Medical Education

"Precision medical education" is the use of tools such as AI to standardize trainees' medical skills and knowledge yet also individualize the delivery and practice of those skills and knowledge. In line with this paradigm, our institution has developed the Adaptive Radiology Interpretation and Education System (ARIES).[59,60] ARIES is a Bayesian network where trainees can select a subsystem network (such as spine), input imaging and clinical features (such as T1 intensity, diffusion restriction, and age), and receive a differential diagnosis from expert-derived prior probabilities. Probabilities can be computed from radiographic features alone or with radiographic and clinical data, allowing for a nuanced discussion of diagnosis.

For example, if a patient presents with deficits localized to the cervical spinal cord and imaging reveals a single, homogeneously enhancing and expansile intramedullary lesion that does not have diffusion restriction, the differential diagnosis includes ependymoma and astrocytoma (**Fig. 2**). Although imaging features may favor ependymoma, clinical features such as patient age (younger than 30 years) and gender (male) may favor astrocytoma.

Bayesian networks can be integrated with lesion and anatomic segmentation methods and teaching files. These AI-augmented teaching databases can create learning profiles for individual trainees, keep track of progress, and recommend relevant cases for trainees to achieve learning milestones.[20,61] Studies have shown that AI can assist education through optimally spaced repetition[62] and the same may be true for practice case–based learning and high-fidelity simulation training. Because there is little data that AI can improve student outcomes, validation studies must be performed. Notably, AI may hold utility even for people who do not initially benefit from AI (**Fig. 3**). For example, AI may enable adaptive learning for people who do worse or not sufficiently well when using AI and assist in adapting itself until the trainee benefits.

It is important to emphasize that the usage of AI systems is not to scrutinize trainees or replace educators. Instead, AI should be used as a support to trainees and a supplement to teachers as medicine progresses toward precision education.

Multimodal Integration

Combining multiple imaging modalities improves everyday clinical diagnosis, progression tracking, and prognostication. Ongoing studies aim to apply similar models and architectures, trained on multiple forms of data, to track progress and predict prognosis for many chronic diseases.

Multiple sclerosis

Diagnosis of MS incorporates detection of lesions from neurologic examinations and imaging. Such correlation benefits from conventional to advanced imaging sequences.[29] ML tools can integrate magnetization-prepared rapid gradient echo, magnetization-prepared 2 rapid gradient echo, and three-dimensional FLAIR and double inversion recovery (DIR) for the detection of MS lesions.[31] In addition, joining NNs with graph theory approaches can classify distinct clinical subtypes of MS based on MR and diffusion tensor imaging (DTI).[63]

Integrated data may not only improve MS diagnosis but also management. Treatment

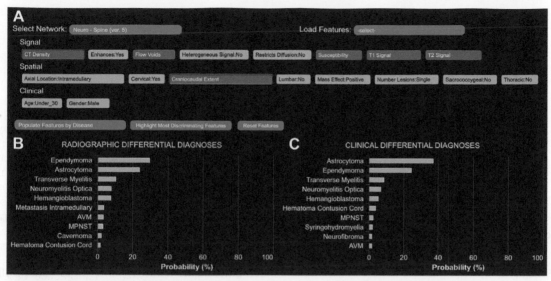

Fig. 2. The Adaptive Radiology Interpretation and Education System (ARIES) distinguishes between ependymoma and astrocytoma in the spine network. (*A*) Features based on signal, spatial, and clinical information are selected by the trainee in blue. Unselected features are gray and the most differentiating unanswered features are highlighted in orange. Differential diagnoses by (*B*) imaging features only versus (*C*) a combination of clinical and imaging features are derived from manually selected features (*A*). Probabilities are calculated by a naïve Bayes network.

response to disease-modifying biological therapy such as natalizumab can be predicted with high-dimensional ML models.[64] In the future, AI used in longitudinal MR imagings[65] may be integrated with clinical assessment, cerebrospinal fluid biomarkers, and genetic susceptibility for better diagnosis and management of MS (**Fig. 4**).

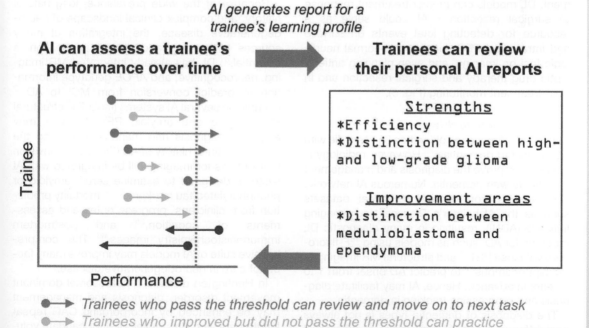

Fig. 3. Feedback loop framework for longitudinal AI-augmented precision education.

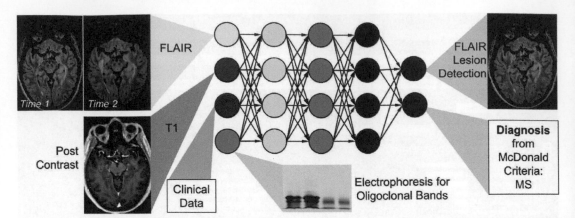

Fig. 4. Model of multimodal integration of AI in diagnosis and assessment of disease progression in multiple sclerosis.

Epilepsy

Diagnosis and management in epilepsy may also be augmented with AI. Several SVMs have been shown to detect abnormalities in temporal lobe epilepsy with cortical morphology on T1w MR imaging and diffusion changes on DTI with kurtosis, mean diffusivity, and fractional anisotropy.[66,67] We envision a future AI system to integrate neuroimaging with DL/ML tools for electroencephalography (EEG) event classification[68–70] and DL-based wearable devices.[71]

Since timely anticonvulsant therapy is essential for improved outcomes in epilepsy,[72] future AI may be applied to both diagnosis and management. DL models can predict treatment response to surgical resection.[73] AI could serve as a resource for detecting ictal events on surface and intracranial EEG, localizing abnormal neurologic foci on imaging, and even planning antiepileptic drug therapy and surgical resection and in post-treatment monitoring (**Fig. 5**).[74]

Neurodegenerative disease

About 1 in 3 Americans older than 85 years die with AD or related dementias.[75] However, radiology is poised to improve the diagnosis and management of patients with dementia. Numerous AI networks have trained from large longitudinal datasets such as the Alzheimer's Disease Neuroimaging Initiative (ADNI), resulting in many diagnostic DL methods for AD, such as models using ^{18}F-fluorodeoxyglucose PET[76] and structural MR imaging of the hippocampus[77] to predict AD onset from 1 to 6 years in advance. Hence, AI may facilitate diagnosis and progression tracking in dementia.

The diagnosis of dementia types is not always straightforward and AI may assist in differential diagnosis. SVMs can distinguish AD from Lewy body and Parkinson dementia.[78] Similarly, CNNs can differentiate mild cognitive impairment (MCI) and AD.[79] In addition to diagnosis, progression, and prognosis, integrative AI can also probe neurobiology. New ML techniques such as Subtype and Stage Inference (SuStaIn) have provided novel neuroimaging and genotype data-driven classifications of diagnostic subtypes and progressive stages for AD and frontotemporal dementia (FTD). SuStaIn has localized distinct regional hotspots for atrophy in different forms of familial FTD caused by mutations in genes including *C9orf72*, *GRN*, and *MAPT*.[80] Thus, neuroimaging AI tools may encourage novel neurobiological discoveries.

Because of the wide prevalence, long natural history, and complex clinical landscape of neurodegenerative disease, the integration of many sources of imaging and clinical information is essential.[81] DL has already integrated MR imaging, neurocognitive, and *APOE* genotype information to predict conversion from MCI to AD.[82] Combining several AI systems (including structural MR imaging and amyloid PET) together may augment diagnosis and management along the complex natural history of AD (**Fig. 6**). We envision that AI tools for imaging will be integrated with AI systems designed to examine serum amyloid or phosphorylated tau markers,[83,84] mortality prediction from clinicians' progress notes and assessments of cognition,[85] and postmortem immunohistochemistry images.[86] This comprehensive suite of AI models may improve many facets of care in neurodegenerative disease.

In Huntington disease, an autosomal dominant movement disorder, diagnosis and management may be enhanced by incorporating CAG repeat length data with NNs developed for caudate volumetry,[45] objective gait assessment,[87] and EEG.[88,89] Such multipronged approaches may

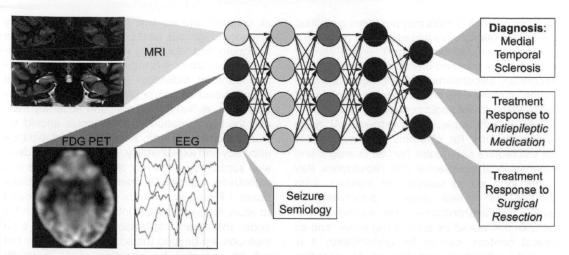

Fig. 5. Model of multimodal integration in diagnosis and management of epilepsy. Bilateral mesial temporal sclerosis demonstrates increased signal and volume loss in hippocampal MR imaging, temporal lobe hypometabolism on ^{18}F-fluorodeoxyglucose (FDG) PET and ictal events on EEG.

improve risk stratification, progression monitoring, and clinical management in patients and families.

Towards a Generalized Neuroimaging Artificial Intelligence

Currently in its infancy stages, AI has potential to support neuroradiological diagnosis in drafting reports for radiologists to review. Yet, differential diagnosis in neuroradiology is particularly complex. A "generalized" AI capable of end-to-end

neuroimaging diagnosis (where inputs are imaging studies and the output is a draft report) will require abilities to extract imaging features, process clinical notes, parcellate neuroanatomy, construct differential diagnoses, recognize potential sources of artifact, compare with prior studies, and more. Future development of more inclusive AI systems may go beyond imaging quantification and incorporate studies from nuclear medicine, electrophysiology, laboratory findings, and clinical data.

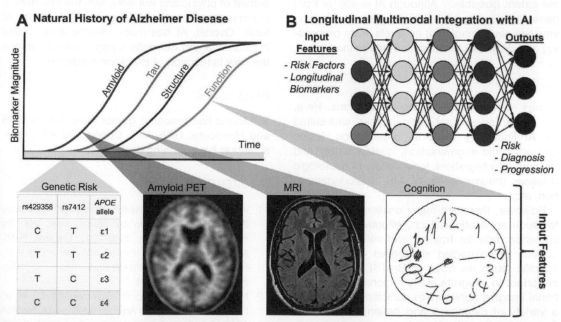

Fig. 6. Model of multimodal integration of AI for diagnosis and management in AD. (A) Natural history of AD (adapted from[81]). (B) AI-enabled multimodal integration of input features for longitudinal (re)assessment of risk, diagnosis, and progression.

Such generalized AI tools may put these quantified numbers in perspective and eventually generate a comprehensive radiology report, which can be used to make informed clinical decisions in multi-disciplinary discussions. This will require the integration of many different AI systems trained on a vast wealth of neurologic conditions.

Even if achievable, an end-to-end AI diagnostic resource for clinicians and radiologists will still require substantial human oversight and supervision. It is essential that radiologists stay in the loop on all aspects of imaging, from ordering the correct study to supervising its quality and interpretation. The significance of the question asked by an imaging order, and its clinical context, cannot be understated; it is currently difficult to imagine an AI algorithm able to account for the unique context in which an imaging study is ordered for a patient. In addition, as data specialists, radiologists must provide continual, real-time feedback to update the AI system.[90] This enables physicians to serve as part of the "checks and balances" between human and machine.

Current research trends (see **Fig. 1**) do suggest that early prototypes of such a generalized AI are on the horizon. These proposed integrated and knowledgeable AIs build on existing multiorgan AI systems.[91,92] An effective generalized AI should also promote precision medical education and produce information that is "interpretable" and "explainable" for trainees and physicians alike to the extent possible.[93] Although AI is still far from generalized utility, it holds promise to one day improve neuroimaging at all levels, from processing and diagnosis to education and management.

DISCUSSION

AI has myriad neuroimaging applications. Here, we presented several clinical tasks well-suited for AI (including workflow organization, lesion and anatomic segmentation, quality, safety and multimodal integration), for a variety of neurologic diseases (trauma, epilepsy, MS, neurodegeneration, etc.)

However, there are many challenges facing AI for such applications. First, effective AI requires immense data for training and validation. Many current neuroimaging databases are disease-specific (such as ADNI or BraTS), so it will be important to integrate many regional and international imaging networks to sufficiently train AI for a variety of diagnoses and patient populations. Second, multimodal AI tools are computationally costly, and significant investment in infrastructure is required. Third, not only are current AI systems

all uniquely trained but they are also uniquely designed. Rigorous best practices are required in designing and validating AI networks. For multi-modal integration, it is important to assess the effect of each individual input modality toward output detection and/or diagnosis. Hence, strategies such as "leave-one-out" and accuracy metrics for segmentation and diagnosis should be standardized.[94] Fourth, clinical AI must balance accuracy and explainability. Although clinical decision support systems rely on known features and algorithms, current DL methods are still "black boxes." Rigorous methods should be developed to allow for better model introspection, which fall under the recent explainable AI methods; such methods are beyond the scope of this review but will be essential for adoption of AI in health care.[93,95] Indeed, our group has demonstrated that an AI system combining deep learning and Bayesian networks for brain MRI can generate accurate and interpretable output such as differential diagnoses and lesion characteristics across a variety of neurological disorders.[96,97] Fifth, adoption will depend on demonstrated improvement in patient outcomes and radiologist efficiency and collective agreement on the benefits of AI. This will require studies designed similar to clinical drug trials for trainees and attending radiologists. Akin to phase 4 studies, AI tools must be monitored after adoption to fine-tune algorithms. Sixth, physicians must be trained in using AI to recommend such algorithm adjustments. It is likely that an emerging subset of physicians will work with the informatics community to continually monitor and update AI tools. Overall, AI has many diverse applications in neuroimaging currently being validated across the new landscape of precision medicine.

DISCLOSURE

S. Mohan has research grants from Galileo CDS and Novocure, USA. M.T. Duong and A.M. Rauschecker have nothing to disclose.

REFERENCES

1. World Health Organization. Global health estimates 2015: Disease burden by cause, age, sex, by country and by region, 2000–2015. Geneva. 2016. Available at: http://www.who.int/healthinfo/global_burden_disease/estimates/en/index1.html. Accessed August 3, 2019.

2. Hassabis D, Kumaran D, Summerfield C, et al. Neuroscience-Inspired Artificial Intelligence. Neuron 2017;95:245–58.

3. Kriegeskorte N. Deep neural networks: a new framework for modeling biological vision and brain

information processing. Annu Rev Vis Sci 2015;1: 417–46.

4. Erickson BJ, Korfiatis P, Akkus Z, et al. Machine learning for medical imaging. Radiographics 2017; 37:505–15.

5. Kohli M, Prevedello LM, Filice RW, et al. Implementing machine learning in radiology practice and research. AJR Am J Roentgenol 2017;208:754–60.

6. Viera S, Pinaya WHL, Mechelli A. Using deep learning to investigate the neuroimaging correlates of psychiatric and neurological disorders: Methods and applications. Neurosci Biobehav Rev 2017; 74(A):58–75.

7. Zaharchuk G, Gong E, Wintermark M, et al. Deep learning in neuroradiology. AJNR Am J Neuroradiol 2018. https://doi.org/10.3174/ajnr.A5543.

8. Rudie JD, Rauschecker AM, Bryan RN, et al. Emerging applications of artificial intelligence in neuro-oncology. Radiology 2019;290(3):607–18.

9. Hornik K, Stinchcombe M, White H. Multilayer feedforward networks are universal approximators. Neural Network 1989;2(5):359–66.

10. Chowdhury FA, Nashef L, Elwes RD. Misdiagnosis in epilepsy: a review and recognition of diagnostic uncertainty. Eur J Neurol 2008;15:1034–42.

11. Solomon AJ, Bourdette DN, Cross AH, et al. The contemporary spectrum of multiple sclerosis misdiagnosis: A multicenter study. Neurology 2016;87: 1393–9.

12. Tarnutzer AA, Lee SH, Robinson KA, et al. ED misdiagnosis of cerebrovascular events in the era of modern neuroimaging: A meta-analysis. Neurology 2017;88:1468–77.

13. Lees KR, Bluhmki E, von Kummer R, et al. Time to treatment with intravenous alteplase and outcome in stroke: an updated pooled analysis of ECASS, ATLANTIS, NINDS, and EPITHET trials. Lancet 2010;375:1695–703.

14. Saver JL, Goyal M, van der Lugt A, et al. Time to treatment with endovascular thrombectomy and outcomes from ischemic stroke: a meta-analysis. JAMA 2016;316:1279–88.

15. Chen MC, Ball RL, Yang L, et al. Deep learning to classify radiology free-text reports. Radiology 2017;286(3):845–52.

16. Winkel DJ, Heye T, Weikert TJ, et al. Evaluation of an AI-based detection software for acute findings in abdominal computed tomography scans: toward an automated work list prioritization of routine CT examinations. Invest Radiol 2019;54(1):55–9.

17. Steinkamp JM, Chambers CM, Lalevic D, et al. Automated organ-level classification of freetext pathology reports to support a radiology follow-up tracking engine. Radiol Artif Intell 2019;1(5): e180052.

18. Arbabshirani MR, Fornwalt BK, Mongelluzzo GJ, et al. Advanced machine learning in action:

identification of intracranial hemorrhage on computed tomography scans of the head with clinical workflow integration. NPJ Digit Med 2018;1:9.

19. Agarwal V, Bump GM, Heller MT, et al. Resident case volume correlates with clinical performance: finding the sweet spot. Acad Radiol 2019;26: 136–40.

20. Duong MT, Rauschecker AM, Rudie JD, et al. Artificial intelligence for precision education in radiology. Br J Radiol 2019;92:20190389.

21. McCoy DB, Dupont SM, Gros C, et al. Convolutional neural network–based automated segmentation of the spinal cord and contusion injury: deep learning biomarker correlates of motor impairment in acute spinal cord injury. AJNR Am J Neuroradiol 2019; 40(4):37–44.

22. Sharma B, Venugopalan K. Classification of hematomas in brain CT images using neural network. 2014 International Conference on Issues and Challenges in Intelligent Computing Techniques (ICICT). https://doi.org/10.1109/ICICICT.2014. 6781250. Ghaziabad (India), February 7, 2014.

23. Chang PD, Kuoy E, Grinband J, et al. Hybrid 3D/2D Convolutional Neural Network for Hemorrhage Evaluation on Head CT. AJNR Am J Neuroradiol 2018; 39(9):1609–16.

24. Stone JR, Wilde EA, Taylor BA, et al. Supervised learning technique for the automated identification of white matter hyperintensities in traumatic brain injury. Brain Inj 2016;30:1458–68.

25. Achrol AS, Rennert RC, Anders C, et al. Brain metastases. Nat Rev Dis Primers 2019;5. https://doi.org/ 10.1038/s41572-018-0055-y.

26. Grøvik E, Yi D, Iv M, et al. Deep learning enables automatic detection and segmentation of brain metastases on multisequence MRI. J Magn Reson Imaging 2019. https://doi.org/10.1002/jmri.26766.

27. Charron O, Lallement A, Jarnet D, et al. Automatic detection and segmentation of brain metastases on multimodal MR images with a deep convolutional neural network. Comput Biol Med 2018;95:43–54.

28. Liu Y, Stojadinovic S, Hrycushko B, et al. A deep convolutional neural network-based automatic delineation strategy for multiple brain metastases stereotactic radiosurgery. PLoS One 2017;12(10): e0185844.

29. Thompson AJ, Banwell BL, Barkhof F, et al. Diagnosis of multiple sclerosis: 2017 revisions of the McDonald criteria. Lancet Neurol 2018;17(2): 162–73.

30. Yoo Y, Tang LY, Brosch T, et al. Deep learning of joint myelin and T1w MRI features in normal-appearing brain tissue to distinguish between multiple sclerosis patients and healthy controls. Neuroimage Clin 2018;17:169–78.

31. Fartaria MJ, Bonnier G, Roche A, et al. Automated detection of white matter and cortical lesions in early

stages of multiple sclerosis. J Magn Reson Imaging 2016;43:1445–64.

32. Lao Z, Shen D, Liu D, et al. Computer-assisted segmentation of white matter lesions in 3D MR images using support vector machine. Acad Radiol 2008; 15:300–13.

33. Bilello M, Doshi J, Nabavizadeh SA, et al. Correlating cognitive decline with white matter lesion and brain atrophy: magnetic resonance imaging measurements in Alzheimer's disease. J Alzheimers Dis 2015;48:987–94.

34. Rachmadi MF, Valdés-Hernández MDC, Agan MLF, et al. Segmentation of white matter hyperintensities using convolutional neural networks with global spatial information in routine clinical brain MRI with none or mild vascular pathology. Comput Med Imaging Graph 2018;66:28–43.

35. Duong MT, Rudie JD, Wang J, et al. Convolutional neural network for automated FLAIR lesion segmentation on clinical brain MR imaging. AJNR Am J Neuroradiol 2019;40(8):1282–90.

36. Donald JJ, Barnard SA. Common patterns in 558 diagnostic radiology errors. J Med Imaging Radiat Oncol 2012;56(2):173–8.

37. Waite S, Scott J, Gale B, et al. Interpretive Error in Radiology. AJNR Am J Roentgenol 2017;208(4): 739–49.

38. Novosad P, Fonov V, Collins DL, et al. Accurate and robust segmentation of neuroanatomy in T1-weighted MRI by combining spatial priors with deep convolutional neural networks. Hum Brain Mapp 2019. https://doi.org/10.1002/hbm.24803.

39. Wachinger C, Reuter M, Klein T. DeepNAT: deep convolutional neural network for segmenting neuroanatomy. Neuroimage 2018;170:434–45.

40. Li S, Shi F, Pu F, et al. Hippocampal shape analysis of alzheimer disease based on machine learning methods. AJNR Am J Neuroradiol 2007;28(7): 1339–45.

41. Tsao S, Gajawelli N, Zhou J, et al. Feature selective temporal prediction of Alzheimer's disease progression using hippocampus surface morphometry. Brain Behav 2017;7(7):e00733.

42. Ataloglou D, Dimou A, Zarpalas D, et al. Fast and precise hippocampus segmentation through deep convolutional neural network ensembles and transfer learning. Neuroinformatics 2019. https://doi.org/10.1007/s12021-019-09417-y.

43. Xie L, Wisse LEM, Pluta J, et al. Automated segmentation of medial temporal lobe subregions on in vivo T1-weighted MRI in early stages of Alzheimer's disease. Hum Brain Mapp 2019;40(12):3431–51.

44. Hobbs NZ, Henley SM, Wild EJ, et al. Automated quantification of caudate atrophy by local registration of serial MRI: evaluation and application in Huntington's disease. Neuroimage 2009;47(4): 1659–65.

45. Rizk-Jackson A, Stoffers D, Sheldon S, et al. Evaluating imaging biomarkers for neurodegeneration in pre-symptomatic Huntington's disease using machine learning techniques. Neuroimage 2011;56(2): 788–96.

46. Brown AD, Marotta TR. A Natural Language Processing-based Model to Automate MRI Brain Protocol Selection and Prioritization. Acad Radiol 2017;24(2):160–6.

47. Kang H, Hii M, Le M, et al. Gadolinium deposition in deep brain structures: relationship with dose and ionization of linear gadolinium-based contrast agents. AJNR Am J Neuroradiol 2018;39: 1597–603.

48. Gong E, Pauly JM, Wintermark M, et al. Deep learning enables reduced gadolinium dose for contrast-enhanced brain MRI. J Magn Reson Imaging 2018;48:330–40.

49. Kleesiek J, Morshuis JN, Isensee F, et al. Can Virtual Contrast Enhancement in Brain MRI Replace Gadolinium?: A Feasibility Study. Invest Radiol 2019; 54(10):653–60.

50. Chen H, Zhang Y, Zhang W, et al. Low-dose CT via convolutional neural network. Biomed Opt Express 2017;8:679–94.

51. Kang E, Min J, Ye JC. A deep convolutional neural network using directional wavelets for low-dose X-ray CT reconstruction. Med Phys 2017;44:1–32.

52. Chen KT, Gong E, Macruz FBdC, et al. Ultra–low-dose 18F-florbetaben amyloid PET imaging using deep learning with multi-contrast MRI inputs. Radiology 2018;290(3):249–56.

53. Chen KT, Schürer M, Ouyang J, et al. Quantitative brain imaging using integrated PET/MRI Investigating the optimal method to generalize an ultra-low-dose amyloid PET/MRI deep learning network across scanner models. J Cereb Blood Flow Metab 2019;39(1S):113–4.

54. Kaplan S, Zhu YM. Full-dose PET image estimation from low-dose PET image using deep learning: a pilot study. J Digit Imaging 2018. https://doi.org/10.1007/s10278-018-0150-3.

55. Xiang L, Qiao Y, Nie D, et al. Deep auto-context convolutional neural networks for standard-dose PET image estimation from low-dose PET/MRI. Neurocomputing 2017;267:406–16.

56. Ouyang J, Chen KT, Gong E, et al. Ultra-low-dose PET reconstruction using generative adversarial network with feature matching and task-specific perceptual loss. Med Phys 2019. https://doi.org/10.1002/mp.13626.

57. Zhu B, Liu JZ, Cauley SF, et al. Image reconstruction by domain-transform manifold learning. Nature 2018;555:487–92.

58. Sreekumari A, Shanbhag D, Yeo D, et al. A deep learning–based approach to reduce rescan and recall rates in clinical MRI examinations. AJNR Am

J Neuroradiol 2019. https://doi.org/10.3174/ajnr. A5926.

59. Chen P-H, Botzolakis E, Mohan S, et al. Feasibility of streamlining an interactive Bayesian-based diagnostic support tool designed for clinical practice. In: Zhang J, Cook TS, editors. Proceedings of SPIE Medical Imaging. San Diego (CA), April 5, 2016. pp.97890C.

60. Duda JT, Botzolakis E, Chen P-H, et al. Bayesian network interface for assisting radiology interpretation and education. In: Zhang J, Chen P.-H, editors. Proceedings of SPIE Medical imaging. Houston (TX), March 6, 2018. pp.26.

61. Chen P-H, Loehfelm TW, Kamer AP, et al. Toward data-driven radiology education-early experience building multi-institutional academic trainee interpretation log database (MATILDA). J Digit Imaging 2016;29:638–44.

62. Tabibian B, Upadhyay U, De A, et al. Enhancing human learning via spaced repetition optimization. Proc Natl Acad Sci U S A 2019;116(10):3988–93.

63. Marzullo A, Kocevar G, Stamile C, et al. Classification of multiple sclerosis clinical profiles via graph convolutional neural networks. Front Neurosci 2019;12:594.

64. Kanber B, Nachev P, Barkhof F, et al. High-dimensional detection of imaging response to treatment in multiple sclerosis. NPJ Digit Med 2019;2:49.

65. Arani LA, Hosseini A, Asadi F, et al. Intelligent computer systems for multiple sclerosis diagnosis: a systematic review of reasoning techniques and methods. Acta Inform Med 2018;26(4):258–64.

66. Rudie JD, Colby JB, Salamon N. Machine learning classification of mesial temporal sclerosis in epilepsy patients. Epilepsy Res 2015;117:63–9.

67. Del Gaizo J, Mofrad N, Jensen JH, et al. Using machine learning to classify temporal lobe epilepsy based on diffusion MRI. Brain Behav 2017;7: e00801.

68. Ullah I, Hussain M, Qazi E-u-H, et al. An automated system for epilepsy detection using EEG brain signals based on deep learning approach. Expert Syst Appl 2018;107:61–71.

69. Zhou M, Tian C, Cao R, et al. Epileptic seizure detection based on EEG signals and CNN. Front Neuroinformatics 2018;12:95.

70. Hossain MS, Amin SU, Alsulaiman M, et al. Applying deep learning for epilepsy seizure detection and brain mapping visualization. ACM Trans Multimed Comput Comm Appl 2019;15(1s):10.

71. Kiral-Kornek I, Roy S, Nurse E, et al. Epileptic seizure prediction using big data and deep learning: toward a mobile system. EBioMedicine 2018;27: 103–11.

72. Krumholz A, Wiebe S, Gronseth GS, et al. Evidence-based guideline: management of an unprovoked first seizure in adults: report of the guideline

development subcommittee of the American Academy of Neurology and the American Epilepsy Society. Neurology 2015;84(16):1705–13.

73. Gleichgerrcht E, Munsell B, Bhatia S, et al. Deep learning applied to whole brain connectome to determine seizure control after epilepsy surgery. Epilepsia 2018;59:1643–54.

74. Nagaraj V, Lee S, Krook-Magnuson E, et al. The Future of Seizure Prediction and Intervention: Closing the loop. J Clin Neurophysiol 2015;32(3): 194–206.

75. Alzheimer's Association. 2019 Alzheimer's Disease Facts and Figures. Alzheimers Dement 2019;15(3): 321–87.

76. Ding Y, Sohn JH, Kawczynski MG, et al. A deep learning model to predict a diagnosis of alzheimer disease by using 18F-FDG PET of the brain. Radiology 2019;290(2):456–64.

77. Li H, Habes M, Wolk DA, et al. A deep learning model for early prediction of Alzheimer's disease dementia based on hippocampal magnetic resonance imaging data. Alzheimers Dement 2019;1–19. https://doi.org/10.1016/j.jalz.2019.02.007.

78. Katako A, Shelton P, Goertzen AL, et al. Machine learning identified an Alzheimer's disease-related FDG-PET pattern which is also expressed in Lewy body dementia and Parkinson's disease dementia. Sci Rep 2018;8:13236.

79. Basaia S, Agosta F, Wagner L, et al. Automated classification of Alzheimer's disease and mild cognitive impairment using a single MRI and deep neural networks. NeuroImage: Clin 2019;21:101645.

80. Young AL, Marinescu RV, Oxtoby NP, et al. Uncovering the heterogeneity and temporal complexity of neurodegenerative diseases with Subtype and Stage Inference. Nat Commun 2018;9:4273.

81. Jack CR, Knopman DS, Jagust WJ, et al. Update on hypothetical model of Alzheimer's disease biomarkers. Lancet Neurol 2013;12(2):207–16.

82. Spasov S, Passamonti L, Duggento A, et al. A parameter-efficient deep learning approach to predict conversion from mild cognitive impairment to Alzheimer's disease. NeuroImage 2019;189:276–87.

83. Ashton NJ, Nevado-Holgado AJ, Barber IS, et al. A plasma protein classifier for predicting amyloid burden for preclinical Alzheimer's disease. Sci Adv 2019;5(2):eaau7220.

84. Goudey B, Fung BJ, Schieber C, et al. A blood-based signature of cerebrospinal fluid Aβ1-42 status. Sci Rep 2019;9(1):4163.

85. Wang L, Sha L, Lakin JR, et al. Development and validation of a deep learning algorithm for mortality prediction in selecting patients with dementia for earlier palliative care interventions. JAMA Netw Open 2019;2(7):e196972.

86. Tang Z, Chuang KV, DeCarli C, et al. Interpretable classification of Alzheimer's disease pathologies

with a convolutional neural network pipeline. Nat Commun 2019;10:2173.

87. Ye Q, Xia Y, Yao Z. Classification of gait patterns in patients with neurodegenerative disease using adaptive neuro-fuzzy inference system. Comput Math Methods Med 2018;9831252. https://doi.org/10.1155/2018/9831252.

88. Odish OFF, Johnsen K, van Someren P, et al. EEG may serve as a biomarker in Huntington's disease using machine learning automatic classification. Sci Rep 2018;8:16090.

89. de Tommaso M, De Carlo F, Difruscolo O, et al. Detection of subclinical brain electrical activity changes in Huntington's disease using artificial neural networks. Clin Neurophysiol 2003;114(7):1237–45.

90. Jha S, Topol EJ. Adapting to artificial intelligence: radiologists and pathologists as information specialists. JAMA 2016;316(22):2353–4.

91. Kermany DS, Goldbaum M, Cai W, et al. Identifying medical diagnoses and treatable diseases by image-based deep learning. Cell 2018;172:1122–31.

92. Binder T, Tantaoui EM, Pati P, et al. Multi-organ gland segmentation using deep learning. Front Med 2019;6:173.

93. Holzinger A, Langs G, Denk H, et al. Causability and explainability of artificial intelligence in medicine. Wiley Interdiscip Rev Data Min Knowl Discov 2019;9(4):e1312.

94. Walker EA, Petscavage-Thomas JM, Fotos JS, et al. Quality metrics currently used in academic radiology departments: results of the QUALMET survey. Br J Radiol 2017;90:20160827.

95. Tjoa E, Guan C. A Survey on Explainable Artificial Intelligence (XAI): Towards Medical XAI. arXiv 2019;1907:07374v3. Available at: https://arxiv.org/abs/1907.07374.

96. Rauschecker AM, Rudie JD, Xie L, et al. Artificial Intelligence System Approaching Neuroradiologist-level Differential Diagnosis Accuracy at Brain MRI. Radiology 2020;295(3):626–37. https://doi.org/10.1148/radiol.2020190283.

97. Rudie JD, Rauschecker AM, Xie L, et al. Subspecialty-level deep gray matter differential diagnoses with deep learning and Bayesian networks on clinical brain MRI: a pilot study. Radiology: Artificial Intelligence, in press.

Machine Learning Applications for Head and Neck Imaging

Farhad Maleki, PhD[a], William Trung Le, BSc[b], Thiparom Sananmuang, MD[c], Samuel Kadoury, PhD[b,d], Reza Forghani, MD, PhD[a,e,f,g,h],*

KEYWORDS

- Head and neck imaging • Autosegmentation • Classification • Machine learning • Deep learning
- Convolutional neural network • Artificial intelligence • Head and neck cancer

KEY POINTS

- Data from head and neck (HN) imaging alongside clinical data can be used to build predictive models improving noninvasive characterization of HN cancers and other anomalies.
- Machine learning (ML) has shown the potential for building predictive models that lead to improved HN tumor characterization, prediction of treatment response, and survival.
- Successful deployment of ML-based models in a clinical setting will require algorithms based on large-scale studies that encompass various sites and variations enabling the future ability to generalize.

INTRODUCTION

Head and neck (HN) imaging is concerned with the evaluation of disorders affecting the complex structures and spaces of the neck, paranasal sinuses, skull base, and the orbits. Like any other anatomic area, the HN can be affected by a large variety of neoplastic and nonneoplastic disorders. However, the HN is notable for its complex anatomy and the concentration of critical organs in close proximity to one another, making advanced imaging and highly specialized expert

interpretations particularly important for the diagnosis and treatment of different disorders affecting this region. Cross-sectional imaging plays a fundamental role in the evaluation of major disorders affecting the HN.

For the work-up of HN lesions such as HN cancer, imaging can be used to identify tumors and, when appropriate, suggest a differential diagnosis for distinguishing benign from malignant lesions. Furthermore, in HN cancer, one of the most fundamental roles of cross-sectional imaging is to accurately determine the stage of a tumor, including

Funding: R. Forghani is a clinical research scholar (chercheur-boursier clinicien) supported by the Fonds de recherche en santé du Québec (FRQS) and has an operating grant jointly funded by the FRQS and the Fondation de l'Association des radiologistes du Québec (FARQ).

[a] Augmented Intelligence & Precision Health Laboratory (AIPHL), Department of Radiology & Research Institute of the McGill University Health Centre, 5252 Boulevard de Maisonneuve Ouest, Montreal, Quebec H4A 3S5, Canada; [b] Polytechnique Montreal, PO Box 6079, succ. Centre-ville, Montreal, Quebec H3C 3A7, Canada; [c] Department of Diagnostic and Therapeutic Radiology and Research, Faculty of Medicine Ramathibodi Hospital, Ratchathewi, Bangkok 10400, Thailand; [d] CHUM Research Center, 900 St Denis Street, Montreal, Quebec H2X 0A9, Canada; [e] Department of Radiology, McGill University, 1650 Cedar Avenue, Montreal, Quebec H3G1A4, Canada; [f] Segal Cancer Centre, Lady Davis Institute for Medical Research, Jewish General Hospital, 3755 Cote Ste-Catherine Road, Montreal, Quebec H3T 1E2, Canada; [g] Gerald Bronfman Department of Oncology, McGill University, Suite 720, 5100 Maisonneuve Boulevard West, Montreal, Quebec H4A3T2, Canada; [h] Department of Otolaryngology, Head and Neck Surgery, Royal Victoria Hospital, McGill University Health Centre, 1001 boul. Decarie Boulevard, Montreal, Quebec H3A 3J1, Canada
* Corresponding author. Room C02.5821, 1001 Decarie Blvd, Montreal, Quebec H4A 3J1, Canada.
E-mail address: reza.forghani@mcgill.ca

evaluation of deep spaces in the neck that may not be reliably evaluated by clinical physical examination and endoscopy, upstaging the initial clinical assessment when appropriate. After treatment, imaging is an essential diagnostic tool for the surveillance of tumor recurrence or differentiation of tumor recurrence from treatment-related complications.[1] In most North American institutions, contrast-enhanced computed tomography (CT) scans, magnetic resonance (MR) imaging, and to a lesser extent PET are the mainstay advanced imaging modalities used for initial evaluation and follow-up of nonthyroid malignancies of the HN, whereas ultrasonography is typically the first modality used for the evaluation of thyroid lesions.

In current routine clinical practice, evaluation or interpretation of patient diagnostic medical scans is largely qualitative with only limited use of basic quantitative parameters for lesion evaluation and characterization. Cancer staging is performed using the American Joint Committee on Cancer (AJCC) TNM system, which classifies cancers based on the size and extent of the primary tumor (T), involvement of regional lymph nodes (N), and the presence or absence of distant metastases (M).[2–4] Reflecting the AJCC classification, tumor assessment and staging is largely based on a lesion's anatomic extent, although, in its revised classification that came into effect in 2018, the AJCC created a separate staging system for human papillomavirus (HPV)–associated cancers of the oropharynx, incorporating a molecular marker for tumor staging that reflects the distinct clinicopathologic characteristics of this subtype of head and neck squamous cell carcinoma (HNSCC).[4,5] Although delineation of the anatomic extent of a tumor is clearly important, there is little use of the additional complex quantitative features present on patients' diagnostic images, and incorporation of molecular markers is only rudimentary at this time. The current process is also subjective and depends on the radiologist's or radiation oncologist's level of expertise and experience, resulting in variations that may not be optimal for patient care. With the advances made in computational power and software engineering, there is great potential for leveraging this technology for improving or augmenting diagnostic evaluation in head and neck imaging toward the ultimate goal of more precise, personalized therapy.

This article reviews the various applications of machine learning (ML) in HN imaging. The article begins with a brief overview of the traditional radiomic-ML workflow versus deep learning, followed by a review of several applications of ML in HN imaging. Next, it discusses the challenges and opportunities in using ML for HN imaging, followed by a brief summary.

RADIOMICS AND MACHINE LEARNING

There has been long-standing interest in computerized image analysis for diagnostic decision support, but developments have been accelerated and the potential expanded as a result of the impressive advances in computational power and software engineering in the last decade. One area of much interest and research activity is in texture analysis or, more broadly, radiomics. First introduced in the medical literature in 2012 and defined as high-throughput extraction of quantitative imaging features with the intent of creating mineable databases from radiological images, the definition of radiomics was later expanded to "high-throughput extraction of quantitative features that result in the conversion of images into mineable data and the subsequent analysis of these data for decision support."[6–9] Radiomic approaches perceive medical imaging as a rich source for mining quantitative features as opposed to pictures intended solely for visual and subjective interpretation.[6] These image-based quantitative features, which are referred to as radiomics features, can provide important additional information and serve as biomarkers enabling higher-level characterization of lesions such as tumors, including prediction of different clinical or molecular end points of interest that may not be evident using standard subjective interpretation alone. Radiomic features may even be considered as image extracted omics that can be used along with other features, such as clinical, genomic, or proteomic information, to capture a holistic picture of the lesion phenotype under study.[6,10–12]

Machine learning is commonly used for predictive modeling in radiomics.[13,14] ML refers to quantitative algorithms capable of learning a task given data related to that task.[15] A performance measure, which is commonly referred to as an objective function, error function, or loss function, is used to evaluate and guide the learning process. It is important to emphasize that radiomic feature extraction itself does not necessarily require artificial intelligence (AI) or, more specifically, ML; many of the published texture or radiomic studies are based on more traditional and computer vision approaches derived using clearly defined or explicit mathematical formulas designed by experts, collectively referred to as handcrafted or hand-engineered features. However, ML classifiers are particularly useful for performing prediction modeling or classification tasks based on radiomic features, with examples including tumor classification, prediction of treatment response, or survival among a multitude of possible tasks. Also, ML approaches such as convolutional neural networks (CNNs) can also be used for direct image analysis and feature extraction, a process that may be referred to as deep radiomics, as discussed in this article.[11,12]

This article categorizes applications of ML in HN cancers as those using traditional ML and those using deep learning methods. Methods such as linear regression, support vector machine (SVM), and random forest are considered as traditional ML. In contrast, methods using neural networks with more than 3 hidden layers are considered as deep learning methods. **Fig. 1** shows a typical workflow for the application of a traditional handcrafted radiomic feature extraction approach followed by the use of an ML method in HN imaging. This process starts with image acquisition. Then radiomic features are mined during feature extraction. Next, available clinical or biological features (if any) can be added to the set of mined radiomics features. Because the size of the feature set often is larger than the sample size (ie, the number of medical images), feature selection or other dimensionality reduction approaches such as principal component analysis is used to extract a reduced set of features. These features are then used for model building. The performance of the model is assessed using previously unseen data; that is, data not used for training and fine-tuning the model.

Traditional ML methods rely on handcrafted features, which are extracted from images as inputs. These features are often the result of years of independent research but may be redundant and nonoptimal for a given task. Deep learning, which is a subset of ML, can be used to perform image analysis and has the potential to alleviate the need for handcrafted features. Given a large and representative dataset, deep learning methods can automatically extract discriminative features for a given task during model training. **Fig. 2** shows a typical deep learning workflow in radiomics. As discussed in later in this article, CNNs have been applied to various image processing tasks, including object detection, semantic segmentation, and instance segmentation.[16–20] CNN-based classification and segmentation models have been developed for HN imaging.[21,22] **Fig. 3** shows a typical CNN-based classification model. Unlike traditional ML approaches that involve a feature extraction step and use the extracted features for model building, feature extraction is part of the deep learning models. These models often are end-to-end models and are trained to learn the optimal features from data.

In a supervised learning context, a dataset of inputs and their desired outputs (ground truths) are used to build and fine-tune a model. Through an iterative process, a random batch of inputs is selected and fed to the model. The model output, which is a probability distribution for the classes, is then recorded. Next, the error (ie, the difference between the model output and the desired output)

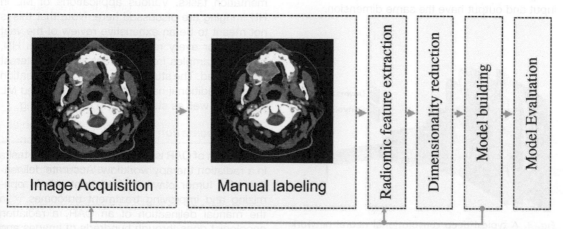

Fig. 1. A typical workflow for the application of traditional handcrafted features and ML methods in radiomics. After acquiring images, they are manually labeled or their region of interest is contoured, depending on the application. Then radiomic features are extracted, most commonly consisting of handcrafted features (variably referred to as texture or radiomic features in the medical literature). Next, dimensionality reduction methods are applied to get a reduced set of features for model building. After training and fine-tuning the model, a collection of sample data that have not been used for building the model is used to evaluate the model performance.

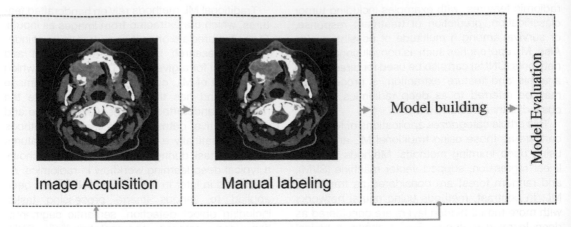

Fig. 2. A typical workflow for deep learning applications in radiomics. After acquiring images, they are manually labeled or contoured, depending on the application. After training and fine-tuning the model, a collection of samples that have not been used for building the model is used to evaluate the model performance. Although in this example the region of interest is manually contoured, with sufficiently large and varied datasets there is potential for deep learning to also perform whole-image analysis, including lesion identification and/or segmentation tasks in an automated or semiautomated fashion.

is measured through a loss function. After that, the model parameters are adjusted using the back-propagation algorithm to minimize the model error.[15] A typical CNN-based model used for image segmentation is shown in **Fig. 4**. This model is similar to the one for classification (see **Fig. 2**). The differences are caused by the nature of the desired output. In classification, an input image needs to be assigned to a category among a predetermined set of options. In contrast, in segmentation, the status of each pixel (voxel) of the input images needs to be determined; therefore, the input and output have the same dimension.

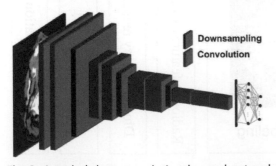

Fig. 3. A typical deep convolutional neural network used for a classification task. A sequence of operators is applied to an input image to produce a dense representation of the input image. This low-dimensional representation is referred to as deep features. These features are then fed to a multilayer perceptron to produce a probability distribution for categories/classes under study.

APPLICATION OF MACHINE LEARNING IN HEAD AND NECK IMAGING

There are several applications of ML that are of clinical interest for the HN. The most common applications include delineation of organ at risk (OAR) or primary tumor for radiation therapy; tumor detection; and tumor phenotyping and precision oncology applications such as prediction of histopathology or molecular phenotype, response to treatment, and survival. These applications often can be categorized as classification or segmentation tasks. Various applications of ML in HN imaging are discussed here. Note that this is not meant to be an exhaustive review of the vast literature or every radiomic or ML study in HN, but key examples from different areas of interest are provided. The studies consist of a combination of more traditional handcrafted radiomics and ML studies as well as studies using deep learning.

Autosegmentation of Organ at Risk

Delineation of OAR is one of the fundamental tasks in a radiation therapy workflow. Accurate delineation of a tumor plays an important role in optimizing and improving treatment outcomes.[23] In the manual delineation of an OAR, a radiation oncologist goes through hundreds of images and tries to delineate the OAR while adjusting various parameters. This task can also be delegated; for example, to a medical physicist, under the supervision of a radiation oncologist. This process is laborious and subject to intraobserver and interobserver variability and is one of the bottlenecks in a

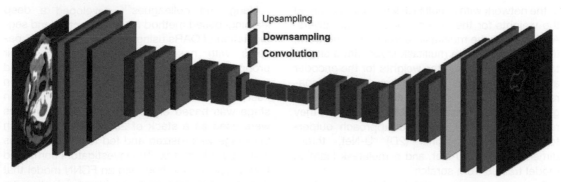

Upsampling
Downsampling
Convolution

Fig. 4. A typical deep convolutional neural network used for an autosegmentation task. A sequence of operators, such as convolutions, upsampling, and downsampling, is applied to the input image to produce a segmentation map as the output.

radiotherapy workflow. ML has been used for tackling this task.[13,21,22,24–31] Atlas-based and deep learning approaches are 2 main categories of methods used for automatic delineation of OAR. Semiautomatic or automatic segmentation, if sufficiently robust, not only has the potential to improve workflow and productivity but also can reduce variations that could result in more consistent contouring and ultimately optimized treatments and outcomes.

Atlas-based methods for autosegmentation of organ at risk or primary tumor

Atlas-based methods for autosegmentation of OAR rely on an image registration method.[29–31] These methods use a library of contoured images, which are referred to as an atlas, to contour a new image. Through an image registration process, the pixels/voxels of a new image are aligned with pixels/voxels of an image from the atlas. Then, by translating the contour of the image in the library (a process called label fusion), a contour for the new image is generated.

Rigid and deformable registration are 2 main approaches for image registration.[32] Rigid registration uses 3 translational and 3 rotational degrees of freedom to overlay 2 images; therefore, all pixels/voxels from 1 image are uniformly transformed or rotated to overlay the other image. This approach often leads to poor results in the presence of patient movement or anatomic changes.[32] In contrast, deformable registration, generates a vector field transformation that maps pixels/voxels from 1 image to pixels/voxels in the other image.[33]

Yang and colleagues[24] proposed a method for autosegmentation of the parotid gland based on atlas registration and SVM. In a longitudinal study of 15 patients with HN cancer, they acquired MR images before radiation therapy and in 3, 6, and

12 months after starting radiation therapy. They used the pretreatment MR imaging and the binary contour for the parotid gland of each patient as an atlas. For each patient, the pretreatment MR imaging was mapped to the posttreatment MR imaging using a deformable image registration approach. Subsequently, the binary contour was transformed using the same mapping. They trained a radial basis function SVM on the pretreatment MR imaging and its transformed contours. The model was used to differentiate the voxels corresponding with the parotid gland from the surrounding tissues on the posttreatment MR images. The output of the autosegmentation system was evaluated against physicians' manual contours. The investigators reported success in parotid segmentation, with an average volume difference between the autosegmentation and the manual contours of 7.98% and 8.12% for the left and right parotid glands, respectively.

Deep learning methods for autosegmentation of organs at risk

Chen and colleagues[22] proposed a CNN architecture using a multitask learning approach aimed at learning multiple tasks at the same time. Then they transferred the learning weights to single-task learning. Their architecture consisted of 3 components: an encoder, a decoder, and a single-task or multitask layer. The encoder contained 4 downsampling layers, and the decoder contained 4 upsampling layers. The output of each encoder layer was concatenated to the input of the corresponding decoder layer. They used 5-by-5 dilated convolutions[34] and residual connections[16] between consecutive layers. Using a life-long learning approach, they trained the autosegmentation system in 3 steps. First, they trained a single-task CNN for segmentation of the spinal cord. Then they substituted the last layer of the network with a multitask layer and preserved the weights for the encoder and decoder layers. After training the multitask segmentation network, they substituted the multitask layer with a single-task layer, preserving the weights for the encoder and decoder layers. The final network was separately trained for the segmentation of 12 HN organs. Using a dataset of 200 HN CT scans, they reported that their proposed approach outperformed two-dimensional (2D) U-Net, three-dimensional (3D) U-Net, and a multitask learning model trained from scratch.

A multiorgan segmentation dataset might be imbalanced because of the variations in the number of annotated organs or differences in the size of organs. Zhu and colleagues[21] developed a 3D CNN model based on the U-Net architecture for the autosegmentation of HN anatomy considering the data imbalances. To address the data imbalance caused by differences in the organ sizes, they adjusted the 3D U-Net architecture. They removed all but 1 of the downsampling layers. They also embedded squeeze-and-excitation layers[35] in the architecture. Also, they proposed and used a hybrid loss function combining Dice coefficient loss and focal loss.[36] To address the data imbalance caused by missing annotations for some anatomic structures, they introduced a class weight into the loss function to assign a higher penalty for the error made in the segmentation of organs with less representation in the dataset. The missing annotations were masked out when calculating the loss function. Using 261 HN CT images from different sites and machines, they trained their model and reported a new and highly effective HN multiorgan segmentation algorithm capable of processing whole-volume CT images.[21]

Tong and colleagues[37] proposed an autosegmentation method for the automatic delineation of 9 HN OARs. The proposed model contains 2 main components: an autoencoder architecture as OARs shape representation model (SRM), and a fully convolutional neural network (FCNN) with a U-shaped architecture similar to that of U-Net.[20] The SRM model, an autoencoder, was trained using segmentation labels and was used as a regularizer when training the FCNN. They used a small dataset of CT images from 32 patients randomly split into a training (22 CT images) and a test set (10 CT images). They reported that their HN autosegmentation method outperformed an atlas-based autosegmentation model[38] that had been the winner of the Medical Image Computing and Computer Assisted Interventions 2015 Head and Neck Auto Segmentation Grand Challenge.[39]

Liang and colleagues[40] developed a deep learning–based method for the detection and segmentation of OARs using CT images from 185 patients with nasopharyngeal carcinoma. Their proposed method had 2 stages: detection and segmentation. The detection stage was based on Fast R-CNN architecture,[41] and the segmentation stage was based on a FCNN.[42] The CT images were used as a stack of 2D axial images. Each 2D image was resized and fed to the network as a 400-by-400 matrix. The investigators compared their proposed method with an FCNN model that directly segmented images without detecting the bounding boxes. They reported that the proposed method achieved significantly higher Dice coefficients compared with the FCNN model. The gain in performance using OAR detection as an intermediary step might be caused by the positions of OARs in CT images being almost consistent; therefore, Fast R-CNN can accurately detect bounding boxes for OARs. Consequently, by eliminating irrelevant information, conducting the segmentation might be an easier task for the model to accomplish.

Deep learning for primary tumor contouring and other advanced radiotherapy applications

In addition to delineation of OARs, studies are also showing the potential value of deep learning for more advanced applications, including automated contouring of primary tumors. In a study by Lin and colleagues,[43] a 3D CNN was trained for automatic primary gross tumor volume (GTV) contouring in patients with nasopharyngeal carcinoma. MR imaging scans from 1021 patients were divided into training, validation, and testing cohorts of 715, 103, and 203 patients, respectively, and GTV contours were defined by consensus of 2 experts. The output from the algorithm was then compared with 8 radiation oncologists in a multicenter evaluation. The AI-generated contours had a high level of accuracy compared with the ground truth (Dice similarity coefficient, 0.79; 2.0-mm difference in average surface distance). Furthermore, during the multicenter evaluation, the use of the AI tool improved contouring accuracy, reduced intraobserver and interobserver variation, and reduced contouring time. In another recent study, by Svecic and colleagues,[44] a deep learning algorithm trained on 337 patients and tested on 50 patients was used as a predictive framework for the evolution of tumor anatomy as well as interfractional dose delivery variations during external beam radiation therapy for HN cancer. Using sequential CT and associated dosimetry data, the probabilistic framework yielded a Dice score of 92% and an overall dose difference of 1.2 Gy in OARs and tumor volume over the multiday treatment course, achieving a 5% reduction in delivered fraction segments.

Phenotype Classification for Head and Neck

The other common type of radiomic and ML studies are those concerned with classification tasks. A classification model is concerned with predicting the most probable category among 2 or several possible options. There are various tasks in HN disorder diagnosis and treatment workflow that can be modeled as a classification problem. Some samples of these tasks are discussed here.

Human papillomavirus prediction

HPV plays an important role in the pathophysiology of HNSCC, representing a distinct clinicopathologic entity and subtype that mainly affects oropharyngeal subsites. The prognosis for patients with HPV-negative HNSCC is poor compared with HPV-positive patients, and their clinical management can differ from their HPV-negative counterparts. HPV status is usually ascertained by using immunohistochemistry for its surrogate marker P16, a protein that hinders cell division, or via direct testing for HPV by in situ hybridization for viral DNA or polymerase chain reaction for HPV oncogene expression. These processes are invasive because they require collecting biospecimens from the patients. HN imaging and ML algorithms have been used for determining HPV status in a noninvasive manner.

Yu and colleagues[45] developed a model to assess HPV status using HN CT imaging. They extracted radiomic features using IBEX software.[46] After a comprehensive feature selection process, a general linear model was built to predict HPV status using the remaining radiomic features. The selected features indicated that HPV-positive tumors are smaller and more spherical compared with HPV-negative tumors. The investigators evaluated the model performance on a public and a private dataset, achieving area under the curve (AUC) values of 0.86667 and 0.91549 for the public and private datasets, respectively.

Buch and colleagues[47] also investigated HPV status prediction using texture features extracted from contrast-enhanced CT images of 40 patients with oropharyngeal squamous cell carcinoma. They identified histogram median, entropy, and GLCM (gray-level co-occurrence matrix) entropy as discriminative features and concluded that radiomics features could be used to predict the HPV status in squamous cell carcinoma. In another study, Vallieres and colleagues[48]

investigated HPV status prediction using 18F-fluorodeoxyglucose PET images of 67 patients with HNSCC. The results of their SVM model supported the feasibility of HPV status prediction for HNSCC. Other studies have also reported variable accuracies for prediction of HNSCC HPV status.[49,50] It is not clear whether ML approaches can reach sufficient accuracy to replace HPV testing, especially given that this testing is done on biopsy specimens and is likely to continue for now. However, a potential role can be foreseen in underserved or under-resourced areas where such testing may not be easy to obtain. Furthermore, the ability to predict HPV status with a relatively high accuracy using noninvasive image analysis and ML suggests the potential value of this approach as a noninvasive biomarker for other tumor phenotypes of interest and precision oncology.

Lymph node classification

Lymph node metastasis and extracapsular lymph node extension are important prognostic factors for HN cancer. Furthermore, more reliable detection of early nodal metastases, especially for oral cavity HNSCCs, has the potential to reduce the need or required extent of neck (nodal) dissection for a subset of those cancers. Kann and colleagues[51] developed a CNN-based model, which they called DualNet, for pretreatment identification of nodal metastasis and extranodal extension using 2875 lymph nodes extracted from 124 patients. The model was then tested on an independent cohort of 131 patients. For the prediction of extranodal extension status, they achieved an AUC value of 0.91 with a negative predictive value of 0.95. For nodal metastasis prediction, they achieved an AUC value of 0.91 with a negative predictive value of 0.82.

Forghani and colleagues[13,52,53] developed an ML approach for the prediction of cervical lymph node metastasis using dual energy CT (DECT) images indirectly by evaluating the radiomic features of the primary HNSCC tumor. They used a retrospective study of 87 patients with histopathology-proven HNSCC. They built a random forest model for nodal status classification that achieved promising results. This study showed that radiomic features of the primary tumor have the potential to be used for nodal status prediction. Their experiments also indicated that multienergy CT scans are superior to single-energy CT scans in predicting cervical lymph node metastasis.

Seidler and colleagues[54] also built random forest and gradient boosting machine models for distinguishing metastatic HNSCC lymph nodes from lymphoma, inflammatory, and normal nodes. They extracted 412 lymph nodes from DECT images of 50 patients. The built models were capable of distinguishing metastatic HNSCC from normal nodes, lymphoma from normal nodes, inflammatory from normal nodes, and malignant from benign lymph nodes. Their results indicated the utility of radiomic feature analysis of DECTs in the identification and histopathologic classification of cervical lymphadenopathy.

Chen and colleagues[55] also reported a hybrid model combining the handcrafted radiomic features and a 3D CNN for classifying lymph nodes as normal, suspicious, or involved. The investigators reported an accuracy of up to 88%. However, the patients did not undergo surgical neck dissection and therefore gold standard pathology proof was not available as ground truth. Studies have also shown the feasibility of evaluating metastatic lymph nodes from thyroid cancer on ultrasonography or CT.[56–58]

ML applications are promising for the evaluation of cervical lymphadenopathy and, if reliable and generalizable algorithms can be developed, have the potential for significant clinical impact. However, there are significant challenges for developing reliable algorithms for this purpose. From the standpoint of algorithm training and ground truth confirmation, it can be challenging to definitively cross-correlate all lymph nodes on imaging with histopathologically confirmed nodes from surgical specimens, especially the smaller nodes that are frequently of the greatest interest from the standpoint of clinical impact. This problem has the potential to introduce both errors and bias. Segmentation and analysis of numerous lymph nodes can also be prohibitively time and labor intensive and, furthermore, many smaller lymph nodes do not have sufficient volume for reliable radiomic analysis. In this regard, much work remains to be done, and a combined approach based on both direct nodal evaluation and indirect predictive modeling based on the analysis of the primary tumor may have the highest likelihood of successful outcome in terms of developing a reliable algorithm with the highest possible accuracy.

Prognosis, risk assessment, and treatment outcome prediction

In an early retrospective study of 72 patients using 2D CT texture analysis, texture features were found to be associated with overall survival in patients with locally advanced HNSCC treated with induction chemotherapy.[59] More recently, Zhang and colleagues[60] developed a model for pretreatment risk assessment of distant metastasis in patients with nasopharyngeal carcinoma using HN MR imaging images. They extracted 2780 radiomics features, among which 7 were selected for building a logistic regression model to classify patients to low risk or high risk of distant metastasis. They trained the model using a retrospective cohort of 123 untreated patients with nonmetastatic status (AUC = 0.827) and validated the trained model using an independent retrospective cohort of 53 patients (AUC = 0.792). The MR images used in this study were acquired from 2 different MR imaging machines and various protocols.

Early studies also suggest the use of MR imaging, CT, and/or PET radiomics and ML for predicting treatment failure or tumor recurrence following radiation and/or chemotherapy for different HN cancers.[49,61,62] Furthermore, pretreatment CT, PET, or MR imaging texture analysis has been used for the prediction of progression-free survival or overall survival in different mucosal HN cancers or thyroid cancer.[63–71]

Thyroid nodule classification

Thyroid cancer is the most prevalent malignancy in the endocrine system. Ultrasonography is commonly used as the first-line diagnostic modality for the detection and characterization of thyroid nodules. Both the acquisition and interpretation of ultrasonography are operator dependent and subjective. The rapid increase in ultrasonography usage has resulted in a significant increase in workload for radiologists, highlighting the need for automatic processing of the resulting data. Consequently, there has been interest in using ML for the detection and diagnosis of thyroid nodules.[72,73]

As an example, Park and colleagues[73] developed a deep learning–based method for the diagnosis of thyroid nodules. Their approach consisted of 3 components. The first component was a fully convolutional network[42] used for the segmentation of a lesion. Each lesion region was manually selected using a bounding box. After conducting segmentation, the tight bounding box for the lesion was selected and expanded by adding some extra margins. A patch of the image corresponding with the expanded bounding box was used as input for the second and third components. For the second component, AlexNet[74] was used to classify 7 ultrasonography features. For the third component, a modified version of GoogLeNet[75] was used to classify the lesion as benign or malignant. The output of the second component was also used as input to the classifier layer used in the third component. They compared the result of the deep learning–based method with the results of an SVM classifier and the manual classifications made by a group of 10 radiologists. They observed that the deep learning–based classifier outperformed the SVM approach. Also, there were no significant differences between the results of the deep learning–based method and the classifications made by the expert radiologists. There are numerous publications exploring the potential of deep learning for thyroid nodule detection or classification, including nodule classification based on standardized risk stratification and classification systems such as the Thyroid Imaging Reporting and Data System.[76–82]

BARRIERS AND CHALLENGES FOR DEEP LEARNING APPLICATIONS IN HEAD AND NECK IMAGING

This article reviews various applications of ML in HN imaging. The research in this area shows promise; however, there are still significant challenges that need to be addressed in order to deploy traditional or deep learning methods in a clinical setting.

A challenge that hinders the clinical application of many ML models as a fully automated system is the imbalanced nature of datasets used for training these models. The accuracy of an ML model could be compromised for patients with uncommon tumor characteristics. Most reported research is considered as proof-of-concept models, because they use small sample sizes often from a single site. Conducting large-scale studies, where the phenotype under study is well represented in the training data, is the next step before the clinical deployment of these methods.

Another source of data imbalance in multiorgan studies is the large difference between the organ sizes. Small structures such as the optic chiasm only compose a small fraction of the whole medical image (0.000,01), which introduces data imbalance.[21] For example, it has been reported that the standard U-Net architecture has difficulty in segmenting organs with small volumes, such as the optic chiasm or optic nerves.[21] Generalized Dice coefficients,[83,84] Tversky,[85] focal loss,[36] sparsity label assignment deep multiinstance learning,[86] and exponential logarithm loss[87] are among the remedies used for dealing with data imbalances. Addressing the data imbalance remains an active area of research.

Deep learning and atlas-based methods are 2 main approaches used for the delineation of OAR. In atlas-based methods, the atlas must include a set of contoured template images that represent the population under study. A deviation from the target population may lead to poor results

for patients with anatomic characteristics that are not well represented in the atlas. Deep learning methods have led to promising results in OAR delineation, which often is the bottleneck in the applications of radiomics. Alleviating this bottleneck will be an important step in providing adaptive treatment planning and personalized radiation therapy.

The output of autosegmentation tools might degrade because of differences in protocols and machinery used for acquiring medical images.[88] Because the error in the delineation of OARs may affect the radiotherapy treatment, a systematic evaluation of available tools through a pilot study is required before putting them into practice. In such a pilot study, a representative subset of the dataset under study should be contoured by experts and be used to evaluate the performance of each tool. Alternatively, autosegmentation can be used to generate an initial segmentation that is reviewed and corrected by an expert. This semi-automated process helps to speed up the contouring process and avoid the error introduced by the autocontouring step. This process also has the advantage of having an expert human as backup, which may also facilitate adoption.

The comparison of various ML applications in HN imaging remains challenging in the lack of large-scale benchmark datasets. This difficulty is more of an issue when evaluating deep learning models, because there are various hyperparameters that may affect the performance of these models. Also, fine-tuning these models is computationally demanding. For example, Chen and colleagues[22] reported that their architecture outperformed the 3D U-Net in the soft Dice and root mean squared error, although the comparison results might not hold when using larger datasets.

In the absence of large-scale medical imaging datasets, transfer learning can be a viable option for achieving performant and generalizable models. For example, the model proposed by Chen and colleagues[22] that used multitask learning and transfer learning outperformed a model with the same architecture trained from scratch.

Annotating medical images requires expertise that is rare and expensive, which is an obstacle for developing large-scale benchmark datasets. To speed up the annotation process, often, each medical image is annotated by a single practitioner. One limitation in such experiments is that the trained model using these datasets might learn the systematic bias or error in the contours. Ideally, the contours should be generated independently by a group of physicians. For each contour, the image and the contour can be used as a training example. This approach is suitable for deep learning applications and can help with alleviating systematic errors in contours generated by a single practitioner. This process can be considered as data augmentation applied to contours. Alternatively, when several physicians have contoured an image, the region encompassing the consensus can be used as the contour for that image.

Assembling large-scale HN imaging datasets is more challenging considering the ethical and legal issues pertaining to patient privacy but could yield superior results. A viable approach for addressing this challenge would be multiorganization collaboration through data sharing platforms with a high level of data security, along with robust anonymization tools for removal of all metadata, possibly supplemented by defacing or equivalent software given the small possibility of surface rendering and facial recognition software for patient identification. Other approaches where the primary data or scan do not leave the institution, such as federated learning, can also be used to enhance privacy protection.

In some applications of deep learning, the lack of sensitivity has been reported.[89] Achieving a sufficiently high sensitivity for the application of interest without sacrificing specificity is an essential requirement for any system with the potential for clinical deployment. A more detailed and general discussion of basic challenges for ML algorithm development, as well as handcrafted radiomics, is beyond the scope of this article but can found in various review articles on the topic.[6,11,12]

SUMMARY

ML has shown the potential to use currently unused data available on patients' medical imaging scans for building predictive models that lead to improved diagnosis and ultimately outcome for patients with different HN disorders, especially HN cancers. Most experiments so far have been proof of concepts and conducted using a small number of samples acquired from a single or a few sites following a single protocol. To be able to deploy these models in a clinical setting, conducting large-scale studies that encompass various sites and protocols, is a requirement. To do so requires developing data aggregation and data sharing pipelines that, while addressing patient privacy concerns, make developing such models possible. If these obstacles can be overcome, ML-based assistive diagnostic tools have the potential to improve both the efficiency and quality of health care, paving the way for more precise and personalized therapies.

REFERENCES

1. Forghani R, Johnson JM, Ginsberg LE. Imaging of Head and Neck Cancer. In: Myers J, Hanna E, Myers EN, editors. Cancer of the head and neck. 5th edition. Philadelphia: Wolters Kluwer; 2017. p. 92–148.

2. Siegel RL, Miller KD, Jemal A. Cancer statistics, 2019. CA A Cancer J Clin 2019;69:7-34. doi:10.3322/caac.21551.

3. Edge SB, Byrd DR, Compton CC, et al. AJCC cancer staging manual. 7th edition. New York: Springer; 2010.

4. Amin MB, Edge S, Greene F, et al. AJCC cancer staging manual. 8th edition. New York: Springer International Publishing; 2017.

5. Chang Z. Will AI improve tumor delineation accuracy for radiation therapy? Radiology 2019;291(3):687–8.

6. Gillies RJ, Kinahan PE, Hricak H. Radiomics: images are more than pictures, they are data. Radiology 2015;278(2):563–77.

7. Sroussi HY, Epstein JB, Bensadoun R-J, et al. Common oral complications of head and neck cancer radiation therapy: mucositis, infections, saliva change, fibrosis, sensory dysfunctions, dental caries, periodontal disease, and osteoradionecrosis. Cancer Med 2017;6(12):2918–31.

8. Kumar V, Gu Y, Basu S, et al. Radiomics: the process and the challenges. Magn Reson Imaging 2012;30(9):1234–48.

9. Lambin P, Rios-Velazquez E, Leijenaar R, et al. Radiomics: extracting more information from medical images using advanced feature analysis. Eur J Cancer 2012;48(4):441–6.

10. Aerts HJ, Velazquez ER, Leijenaar RT, et al. Decoding tumour phenotype by noninvasive imaging using a quantitative radiomics approach. Nat Commun 2014;5:4006.

11. Forghani R, Savadjiev P, Chatterjee A, et al. Radiomics and artificial intelligence for biomarker and prediction model development in oncology. Comput Struct Biotechnol J 2019;17:995–1008.

12. Forghani R. Precision digital oncology: Emerging role of radiomics-based biomarkers and artificial intelligence for advanced imaging and characterization of brain tumors. Radiology: Imaging Cancer 2020;2(4):e190047.

13. Forghani R, Chatterjee A, Reinhold C, et al. Head and neck squamous cell carcinoma: prediction of cervical lymph node metastasis by dual-energy CT texture analysis with machine learning. Eur Radiol 2019;29(11):6172–81.

14. Al Ajmi E, Forghani B, Reinhold C, et al. Spectral multi-energy CT texture analysis with machine learning for tissue classification: an investigation using classification of benign parotid tumours as a testing paradigm. Eur Radiol 2018;28(6):2604–11.

15. Goodfellow I, Bengio Y, Courville A. Deep learning. Cambridge (MA): MIT Press; 2018.

16. He K, Zhang X, Ren S, et al. Deep residual learning for image recognition. Paper presented at: Proceedings of the IEEE conference on computer vision and pattern recognition. Las Vegas (NV), June 26-July 1, 2016.

17. Huang G, Liu Z, Van Der Maaten L, et al. Densely connected convolutional networks. Paper presented at: Proceedings of the IEEE conference on computer vision and pattern recognition. Honolulu (HI), July 22-25, 2017.

18. Pinheiro PO, Lin T-Y, Collobert R, et al. Learning to refine object segments. Paper presented at: European Conference on Computer Vision. Las Vegas (NV), June 26-July 1, 2016.

19. Pinheiro POO, Collobert R, Dollar P. Learning to segment object candidates. Paper presented at: Advances in Neural Information Processing Systems. Montreal (QC), December 7-10, 2015.

20. Ronneberger O, Fischer P, Brox T. U-Net: Convolutional networks for biomedical image segmentation. Paper presented at: International Conference on Medical image computing and computer-assisted intervention. Munich (Germany), October 5-9, 2015.

21. Zhu W, Huang Y, Zeng L, et al. AnatomyNet: Deep learning for fast and fully automated whole-volume segmentation of head and neck anatomy. Med Phys 2019;46(2):576–89.

22. Chan JW, Kearney V, Haaf S, et al. A convolutional neural network algorithm for automatic segmentation of head and neck organs at risk using deep lifelong learning. Med Phys 2019;46(5):2204–13.

23. Ng WT, Lee MCH, Chang ATY, et al. The impact of dosimetric inadequacy on treatment outcome of nasopharyngeal carcinoma with IMRT. Oral Oncol 2014;50(5):506–12.

24. Yang X, Wu N, Cheng G, et al. Automated segmentation of the parotid gland based on atlas registration and machine learning: a longitudinal MRI study in head-and-neck radiation therapy. Int J Radiat Oncol Biol Phys 2014;90(5):1225–33.

25. Wu VWC, Ying MTC, Kwong DLW. Evaluation of radiation-induced changes to parotid glands following conventional radiotherapy in patients with nasopharygneal carcinoma. Br J Radiol 2011;84(1005):843–9.

26. Guidi G, Maffei N, Vecchi C, et al. A support vector machine tool for adaptive tomotherapy treatments: prediction of head and neck patients criticalities. Physica Med 2015;31(5):442–51.

27. Scalco E, Fiorino C, Cattaneo GM, et al. Texture analysis for the assessment of structural changes in parotid glands induced by radiotherapy. Radiother Oncol 2013;109(3):384–7.

28. Eisbruch A, Kim HM, Terrell JE, et al. Xerostomia and its predictors following parotid-sparing irradiation of head-and-neck cancer. Int J Radiat Oncol Biol Phys 2001;50(3):695–704.

29. Kearney V, Chen S, Gu X, et al. Automated landmark-guided deformable image registration. Phys Med Biol 2014;60(1):101.

30. Kearney V, Huang Y, Mao W, et al. Canny edge-based deformable image registration. Phys Med Biol 2017;62(3):966–85.

31. Obeidat M, Narayanasamy G, Cline K, et al. Comparison of different QA methods for deformable image registration to the known errors for prostate and head-and-neck virtual phantoms. Biomed Phys Eng Express 2016;2(6):067002.

32. Fortin D, Basran PS, Berrang T, et al. Deformable versus rigid registration of PET/CT images for radiation treatment planning of head and neck and lung cancer patients: a retrospective dosimetric comparison. Radiat Oncol 2014;9(1):50.

33. Oh S, Kim S. Deformable image registration in radiation therapy. Radiat Oncol J 2017;35(2):101.

34. Yu F, Koltun V. Multi-scale context aggregation by dilated convolutions. arXiv preprint arXiv: 151107122. 2015.

35. Hu J, Shen L, Sun G. Squeeze-and-Excitation Networks. Paper presented at: Proceedings of the IEEE Conference on Computer Vision and Pattern Recognition. Salt Lake City (UT), June 18-22, 2018.

36. Lin T-Y, Goyal P, Girshick R, et al. Focal loss for dense object detection. Paper presented at: The IEEE International Conference on Computer Vision. Venice (Italy), October 22-29, 2017.

37. Tong N, Gou S, Yang S, et al. Fully automatic multi-organ segmentation for head and neck cancer radiotherapy using shape representation model constrained fully convolutional neural networks. Med Phys 2018;45(10):4558–67.

38. Han X, Hoogeman MS, Levendag PC, et al. Atlas-Based Auto-segmentation of Head and Neck CT Images. Paper presented at: Medical Image Computing and Computer-Assisted Intervention–MICCAI. New York, September 6-10, 2008.

39. Mannion-Haworth R, Bowes M, Ashman A, et al. Fully automatic segmentation of head and neck organs using active appearance models. MIDAS J 2016.

40. Liang S, Tang F, Huang X, et al. Deep-learning-based detection and segmentation of organs at risk in nasopharyngeal carcinoma computed tomographic images for radiotherapy planning. Eur Radiol 2019;29(4):1961–7.

41. Ren S, He K, Girshick R, et al. Towards real-time object detection with region proposal networks. IEEE Trans Pattern Anal Mach Intell 2016;39(6):1137–49.

42. Long J, Shelhamer E, Darrell T. Fully convolutional networks for semantic segmentation. Paper

presented at: Proceedings of the IEEE Conference on Computer Vision and Pattern Recognition. Boston (MA), June 7-12, 2015.

43. Lin L, Dou Q, Jin YM, et al. Deep learning for automated contouring of primary tumor volumes by MRI for nasopharyngeal carcinoma. Radiology 2019;291(3):677–86.

44. Svecic A, Roberge D, Kadoury S. Prediction of interfractional radiotherapy dose plans with domain translation in spatiotemporal embeddings. Med Image Anal 2020;64:101728.

45. Yu K, Zhang Y, Yu Y, et al. Radiomic analysis in prediction of Human Papilloma Virus status. Clin Transl Radiat Oncol 2017;7:49–54.

46. Zhang L, Fried DV, Fave XJ, et al. IBEX: an open infrastructure software platform to facilitate collaborative work in radiomics. Med Phys 2015;42(3): 1341–53.

47. Buch K, Fujita A, Li B, et al. Using texture analysis to determine human papillomavirus status of oropharyngeal squamous cell carcinomas on CT. AJNR Am J Neuroradiol 2015;36(7):1343–8.

48. Vallieres M, Kumar A, Sultanem K, et al. FDG-PET image-derived features can determine HPV status in head-and-neck cancer. Int J Radiat Oncol Biol Phys 2013;87(2):S467.

49. Bogowicz M, Riesterer O, Ikenberg K, et al. Computed Tomography Radiomics Predicts HPV status and local tumor control after definitive radiochemotherapy in head and neck squamous cell carcinoma. Int J Radiat Oncol Biol Phys 2017;99(4): 921–8.

50. Haider SP, Mahajan A, Zeevi T, et al. PET/CT radiomics signature of human papilloma virus association in oropharyngeal squamous cell carcinoma. Eur J Nucl Med Mol Imaging 2020. https://doi.org/10.1007/s00259-020-04839-2.

51. Kann BH, Aneja S, Loganadane GV, et al. Pretreatment identification of head and neck cancer nodal metastasis and extranodal extension using deep learning neural networks. Sci Rep 2018; 8(1):14036.

52. Forghani R, De Man B, Gupta R. Dual-energy computed tomography: physical principles, approaches to scanning, usage, and implementation: part 1. Neuroimaging Clin 2017;27(3):371–84.

53. Forghani R, De Man B, Gupta R. Dual-energy computed tomography: physical principles, approaches to scanning, usage, and implementation: part 2. Neuroimaging Clin 2017;27(3):385–400.

54. Seidler M, Forghani B, Reinhold C, et al. Dual-energy CT texture analysis with machine learning for the evaluation and characterization of cervical lymphadenopathy. Comput Struct Biotechnol J 2019;17:1009–15.

55. Chen L, Zhou Z, Sher D, et al. Combining many-objective radiomics and 3D convolutional neural network through evidential reasoning to predict lymph node metastasis in head and neck cancer. Phys Med Biol 2019;64(7):075011.

56. Lee JH, Baek JH, Kim JH, et al. Deep learning-based computer-aided diagnosis system for localization and diagnosis of metastatic lymph nodes on ultrasound: a pilot study. Thyroid 2018;28(10):1332–8.

57. Lee JH, Ha EJ, Kim JH. Application of deep learning to the diagnosis of cervical lymph node metastasis from thyroid cancer with CT. Eur Radiol 2019; 29(10):5452–7.

58. Lee JH, Ha EJ, Kim D, et al. Application of deep learning to the diagnosis of cervical lymph node metastasis from thyroid cancer with CT: external validation and clinical utility for resident training. Eur Radiol 2020;30(6):3066–72.

59. Zhang H, Graham CM, Elci O, et al. Locally advanced squamous cell carcinoma of the head and neck: CT texture and histogram analysis allow independent prediction of overall survival in patients treated with induction chemotherapy. Radiology 2013;269(3):801–9.

60. Zhang L, Dong D, Li H, et al. Development and validation of a magnetic resonance imaging-based model for the prediction of distant metastasis before initial treatment of nasopharyngeal carcinoma: A retrospective cohort study. EBioMedicine 2019;40:327–35.

61. Li S, Wang K, Hou Z, et al. Use of radiomics combined with machine learning method in the recurrence patterns after intensity-modulated radiotherapy for nasopharyngeal carcinoma: a preliminary study. Front Oncol 2018;8:648.

62. Kuno H, Qureshi MM, Chapman MN, et al. CT texture analysis potentially predicts local failure in head and neck squamous cell carcinoma treated with chemoradiotherapy. AJNR Am J Neuroradiol 2017;38(12):2334–40.

63. Mao J, Fang J, Duan X, et al. Predictive value of pretreatment MRI texture analysis in patients with primary nasopharyngeal carcinoma. Eur Radiol 2019; 29(8):4105–13.

64. Cheng NM, Fang YH, Chang JT, et al. Textural features of pretreatment 18F-FDG PET/CT images: prognostic significance in patients with advanced T-stage oropharyngeal squamous cell carcinoma. J Nucl Med 2013;54(10):1703–9.

65. Leijenaar RT, Carvalho S, Hoebers FJ, et al. External validation of a prognostic CT-based radiomic signature in oropharyngeal squamous cell carcinoma. Acta Oncol 2015;54(9):1423–9.

66. Parmar C, Grossmann P, Rietveld D, et al. Radiomic machine-learning classifiers for prognostic biomarkers of head and neck cancer. Front Oncol 2015;5:272.

67. Vallieres M, Kay-Rivest E, Perrin LJ, et al. Radiomics strategies for risk assessment of tumour failure in head-and-neck cancer. Sci Rep 2017;7(1):10117.

68. Park VY, Han K, Lee E, et al. Association between radiomics signature and disease-free survival in conventional papillary thyroid carcinoma. Sci Rep 2019;9(1):4501.

69. Zdilar L, Vock DM, Marai GE, et al. Evaluating the effect of right-censored end point transformation for radiomic feature selection of data from patients with oropharyngeal cancer. JCO Clin Cancer Inform 2018;2:1–19.

70. Zhuo EH, Zhang WJ, Li HJ, et al. Radiomics on multimodalities MR sequences can subtype patients with non-metastatic nasopharyngeal carcinoma (NPC) into distinct survival subgroups. Eur Radiol 2019; 29(10):5590–9.

71. Haider SP, Zeevi T, Baumeister P, et al. Potential Added Value of PET/CT Radiomics for Survival Prognostication beyond AJCC 8th edition staging in oropharyngeal squamous cell carcinoma. Cancers (Basel) 2020;12(7):E1778.

72. Acharya UR, Swapna G, Sree SV, et al. A review on ultrasound-based thyroid cancer tissue characterization and automated classification. Technol Cancer Res Treat 2014;13(4):289–301.

73. Park VY, Han K, Seong YK, et al. Diagnosis of thyroid nodules: performance of a Deep Learning convolutional neural network Model vs. Radiologists. Sci Rep 2019;9(1):1–9.

74. Krizhevsky A, Sutskever I, Hinton GE. ImageNet classification with deep convolutional neural networks. Paper presented at: Advances in Neural Information Processing Systems. Stateline (NV), December 3-8, 2012.

75. Szegedy C, Liu W, Jia Y, et al. Going deeper with convolutions. Paper presented at: Proceedings of the IEEE Conference on Computer Vision and Pattern Recognition2015.

76. Chi J, Walia E, Babyn P, et al. Thyroid nodule classification in ultrasound images by fine-tuning deep convolutional neural network. J Digit Imaging 2017; 30(4):477–86.

77. Li H, Weng J, Shi Y, et al. An improved deep learning approach for detection of thyroid papillary cancer in ultrasound images. Sci Rep 2018;8(1):6600.

78. Song W, Li S, Liu J, et al. Multitask cascade convolution neural networks for automatic thyroid nodule detection and recognition. IEEE J Biomed Health Inform 2019;23(3):1215–24.

79. Ko SY, Lee JH, Yoon JH, et al. Deep convolutional neural network for the diagnosis of thyroid nodules on ultrasound. Head Neck 2019;41(4):885–91.

80. Buda M, Wildman-Tobriner B, Hoang JK, et al. Management of thyroid nodules seen on US images: deep learning may match performance of radiologists. Radiology 2019;292(3):695–701.

81. Akkus Z, Cai J, Boonrod A, et al. A survey of deep-learning applications in ultrasound: artificial intelligence-powered ultrasound for improving clinical workflow. J Am Coll Radiol 2019;16(9 Pt B): 1318–28.

82. Sun C, Zhang Y, Chang Q, et al. Evaluation of a deep learning-based computer-aided diagnosis system for distinguishing benign from malignant thyroid nodules in ultrasound images. Med Phys 2020. https://doi.org/10.1002/mp.14301.

83. Sudre CH, Li W, Vercauteren T, et al. Generalised dice overlap as a deep learning loss function for highly unbalanced segmentations. In: Cardoso J, Arbel T, Carneiro G, et al, editors. Deep learning in medical image analysis and multimodal learning for clinical decision support. Cham (Switzerland): Springer; 2017. p. 240–8.

84. Crum WR, Camara O, Hill DLG. Generalized overlap measures for evaluation and validation in medical image analysis. IEEE Trans Med Imaging 2006; 25(11):1451–61.

85. Salehi SSM, Erdogmus D, Gholipour A. Tversky loss function for image segmentation using 3D fully convolutional deep networks. Paper presented at: International Workshop on Machine Learning in Medical Imaging2017.

86. Zhu W, Lou Q, Vang YS, et al. Deep multi-instance networks with sparse label assignment for whole mammogram classification. Paper presented at: International Conference on Medical Image Computing and Computer-Assisted Intervention2017.

87. Wong KCL, Moradi M, Tang H, et al. 3D segmentation with exponential logarithmic loss for highly unbalanced object sizes. Paper presented at: International Conference on Medical Image Computing and Computer-Assisted Intervention2018.

88. Lee H, Lee E, Kim N, et al. Clinical evaluation of commercial atlas-based auto-segmentation in the head and neck region. Front Oncol 2019;9:239.

89. Wang H, Zhou Z, Li Y, et al. Comparison of machine learning methods for classifying mediastinal lymph node metastasis of non-small cell lung cancer from 18F-FDG PET/CT images. EJNMMI Res 2017;7(1):11.

UNITED STATES POSTAL SERVICE®
Statement of Ownership, Management, and Circulation
(All Periodicals Publications Except Requester Publications)

1. Publication Title	2. Publication Number	3. Filing Date
NEUROIMAGING CLINICS OF NORTH AMERICA	010 – 548	9/18/2020

4. Issue Frequency	5. Number of Issues Published Annually	6. Annual Subscription Price
FEB, MAY, AUG, NOV	4	$397.00

7. Complete Mailing Address of Known Office of Publication (Not printer) (Street, city, county, state, and ZIP+4®)

ELSEVIER INC.
230 Park Avenue, Suite 800
New York, NY 10169

Contact Person
Malathi Samayan

Telephone (Include area code)
91-44-4299-4507

8. Complete Mailing Address of Headquarters or General Business Office of Publisher (Not printer)

ELSEVIER INC.
230 Park Avenue, Suite 800
New York, NY 10169

9. Full Names and Complete Mailing Addresses of Publisher, Editor, and Managing Editor (Do not leave blank)

Publisher (Name and complete mailing address)

DOLORES MELONI, ELSEVIER INC.
1600 JOHN F KENNEDY BLVD. SUITE 1800
PHILADELPHIA, PA 19103-2899

Editor (Name and complete mailing address)

JOHN VASSALLO, ELSEVIER INC.
1600 JOHN F KENNEDY BLVD. SUITE 1800
PHILADELPHIA, PA 19103-2899

Managing Editor (Name and complete mailing address)

PATRICK MANLEY ELSEVIER INC.
1600 JOHN F KENNEDY BLVD. SUITE 1800
PHILADELPHIA, PA 19103-2899

10. Owner (Do not leave blank. If the publication is owned by a corporation, give the name and address of the corporation immediately followed by the names and addresses of all stockholders owning or holding 1 percent or more of the total amount of stock. If not owned by a corporation, give the names and addresses of the individual owners. If owned by a partnership or other unincorporated firm, give its name and address as well as those of each individual owner. If the publication is published by a nonprofit organization, give its name and address.)

Full Name	Complete Mailing Address
WHOLLY OWNED SUBSIDIARY OF REED/ELSEVIER, US HOLDINGS	1600 JOHN F KENNEDY BLVD. SUITE 1800 PHILADELPHIA, PA 19103-2899

11. Known Bondholders, Mortgagees, and Other Security Holders Owning or Holding 1 Percent or More of Total Amount of Bonds, Mortgages, or Other Securities. If none, check box ▶ ☐ None

Full Name	Complete Mailing Address
N/A	

12. Tax Status (For completion by nonprofit organizations authorized to mail at nonprofit rates) (Check one)
The purpose, function, and nonprofit status of this organization and the exempt status for federal income tax purposes:
☒ Has Not Changed During Preceding 12 Months
☐ Has Changed During Preceding 12 Months (Publisher must submit explanation of change with this statement)

PS Form 3526, July 2014 (Page 1 of 4 (see instructions page 4)) PSN: 7530-01-000-9931 PRIVACY NOTICE: See our privacy policy on www.usps.com.

---

13. Publication Title	14. Issue Date for Circulation Data Below
NEUROIMAGING CLINICS OF NORTH AMERICA	MAY 2020

15. Extent and Nature of Circulation		Average No. Copies Each Issue During Preceding 12 Months	No. Copies of Single Issue Published Nearest to Filing Date
a. Total Number of Copies (Net press run)		394	371
b. Paid Circulation (By Mail and Outside the Mail)	(1) Mailed Outside-County Paid Subscriptions Stated on PS Form 3541 (Include paid distribution above nominal rate, advertiser's proof copies, and exchange copies)	293	276
	(2) Mailed In-County Paid Subscriptions Stated on PS Form 3541 (Include paid distribution above nominal rate, advertiser's proof copies, and exchange copies)	0	0
	(3) Paid Distribution Outside the Mails Including Sales Through Dealers and Carriers, Street Vendors, Counter Sales, and Other Paid Distribution Outside USPS®	63	49
	(4) Paid Distribution by Other Classes of Mail Through the USPS (e.g., First-Class Mail®)	0	0
c. Total Paid Distribution (Sum of 15b (1), (2), (3), and (4))	▶	356	325
d. Free or Nominal Rate Distribution (By Mail and Outside the Mail)	(1) Free or Nominal Rate Outside-County Copies included on PS Form 3541	22	31
	(2) Free or Nominal Rate In-County Copies Included on PS Form 3541	0	0
	(3) Free or Nominal Rate Copies Mailed at Other Classes Through the USPS (e.g., First-Class Mail)	0	0
	(4) Free or Nominal Rate Distribution Outside the Mail (Carriers or other means)	0	0
e. Total Free or Nominal Rate Distribution (Sum of 15d (1), (2), (3) and (4))		22	31
f. Total Distribution (Sum of 15c and 15e)	▶	378	356
g. Copies not Distributed (See Instructions to Publishers #4 (page #3))	▶	16	15
h. Total (Sum of 15f and g)	▶	394	371
i. Percent Paid (15c divided by 15f times 100)		94.17%	91.29%

* If you are claiming electronic copies, go to line 16 on page 3. If you are not claiming electronic copies, skip to line 17 on page 3.

16. Electronic Copy Circulation		Average No. Copies Each Issue During Preceding 12 Months	No. Copies of Single Issue Published Nearest to Filing Date
a. Paid Electronic Copies	▶		
b. Total Paid Print Copies (Line 15c) + Paid Electronic Copies (Line 16a)	▶		
c. Total Print Distribution (Line 15f) + Paid Electronic Copies (Line 16a)	▶		
d. Percent Paid (Both Print & Electronic Copies) (16b divided by 16c × 100)	▶		

☒ I certify that 50% of all my distributed copies (electronic and print) are paid above a nominal price.

17. Publication of Statement of Ownership

☒ If the publication is a general publication, publication of this statement is required. Will be printed in the NOVEMBER 2020 issue of this publication. ☐ Publication not required.

18. Signature and Title of Editor, Publisher, Business Manager, or Owner	Date
Malathi Samayan - Distribution Controller *Malathi Samayan*	9/18/2020

I certify that all information furnished on this form is true and complete. I understand that anyone who furnishes false or misleading information on this form or who omits material or information requested on the form may be subject to criminal sanctions (including fines and imprisonment) and/or civil sanctions (including civil penalties).

PS Form 3526, July 2014 (Page 3 of 4) PRIVACY NOTICE: See our privacy policy on www.usps.com.

Moving?

Make sure your subscription moves with you!

To notify us of your new address, find your **Clinics Account Number** (located on your mailing label above your name), and contact customer service at:

Email: journalscustomerservice-usa@elsevier.com

800-654-2452 (subscribers in the U.S. & Canada)
314-447-8871 (subscribers outside of the U.S. & Canada)

Fax number: 314-447-8029

**Elsevier Health Sciences Division
Subscription Customer Service
3251 Riverport Lane
Maryland Heights, MO 63043**

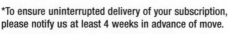

*To ensure uninterrupted delivery of your subscription, please notify us at least 4 weeks in advance of move.

Printed and bound by CPI Group (UK) Ltd, Croydon, CR0 4YY

03/10/2024

01040307-0015